Assertive Community Treatment

of Persons with Severe Mental Illness

**Leonard I. Stein, M.D.
and
Alberto B. Santos, M.D.**

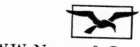

W.W. Norton & Company, Inc.
New York • London

For information about permission to reproduce selections
from this book, write to
Permissions, W. W. Norton & Company, Inc., 500 Fifth Avenue,
New York, NY 10110

The text of this book is composed in New Baskerville
with the display set in Silhouette.
Composition and book design by Paradigm Graphics

Library of Congress Cataloging-in-Publication Data

Stein, Leonard I.
Assertive community treatment of persons with
severe mental illness / Leonard I. Stein and Alberto B. Santos.
p.   cm.
"A Norton Professional Book."
Includes bibliographical references and index.
ISBN 0-393-70258-8 (pbk.)
1. Mentally ill–Services for. 2. Community mental health services
3. Chronically ill–Services for.
I. Santos, Alberto B., 1951–
II. Title.
RC480.53.S74   1998
362.2'2–dc21   97-38893   CIP

W.W. Norton & Company, Inc., 500 Fifth Avenue, New York, N.Y. 10110
http://www.wwnorton.com
W.W. Norton & Company Ltd., 10 Coptic Street, London WC1A 1PU

4   5   6   7   8   9   0

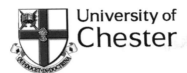

Dedicated to the memory of
Arnold J. Marx, M.D.

Contents

Acknowledgments

The ACT program started at the Mendota Mental Health Institute, Madison, Wisconsin, in the early 1970s. Drs. Leonard Stein, Mary Ann Test, and Arnold Marx were key players in its development. Unfortunately, Dr. Marx died in an accident in 1975; with his death, the field lost a creative thinker and a forceful advocate for the rights of the mentally ill. Drs. Stein and Test, along with many others, lost a friend who added spark to their lives. Dr. Test has been continuously involved in doing cutting-edge research on the ACT model, as well as giving generously of her time in lecturing and consulting on the model; it is difficult for the authors of this volume to conceive of not having Dr. Test as a co-author. Because of time constraints brought about by the unfortunate situation of her parents' ill health and the recent death of her mother, Dr. Test was unable to join us in writing this volume. Although she couldn't join us as an author, much of the material in this volume is a product of her work and thinking, and we are grateful to her for that.

Early in its life, the ACT model struggled for recognition and could have easily faded away had it not been for some key persons and key locations that recognized its value. They not only put the program into practice themselves but were also instrumental in helping others develop their own programs. Dr. William Knoedler and Deborah Allness, MSSW, have dedicated their entire careers to running a superb program in Madison, Wisconsin, as well as traveling all over the United States and to the United Kingdom, providing ongoing consultation, advice, support, and encouragement to scores of fledgling programs, helping them flourish and become models for others to emulate.

The Mental Health Center of Dane County, Inc., located in Madison, Wisconsin, adopted this model as their key program to help the most disabled of the severe and persistently mentally ill in Madison achieve stability and a decent quality of life. The Center operates five ACT programs under the direction of their Program Director, Linda Keys, MSSW; those programs serve over 350 clients. In addition, the ACT programs, along with other Center programs serving persons with serious and persistent mental illness, helped this mental health center develop a comprehensive, integrated, public mental health system that has become internationally recognized and, together with the original ACT program, has been visited by literally hundreds of mental health professionals, administrators, and politicians from all over the world. This Center, like the original program, has served as a beacon and an inspiration to scores of others who have subsequently developed the ACT model. Dr. Ronald Diamond, Medical Director of the Center, has been an absolutely essential figure in both the development of the Center's ACT programs and the comprehensive system of care.

Daniel McCarthy and Ann Detrick were key figures in helping Rhode Island be a leader in utilizing ACT programs to help the severe and persistently mentally ill improve their lives and enabling the state system to move away from institutional care for this population. James Haveman and Tom Plum played a major role in helping the state of Michigan accomplish the same thing. The work of Neil Meisler was instrumental in the development of ACT programs in two states, Delaware and South Carolina.

We are indebted to Linda Keys, Jackie Shivers and her ACT team, David Delap and his ACT team, all of the Mental Health Center of Dane County, Inc., for generously giving their time to be interviewed.

The Mental Health Center of Dane County, Inc., and the state of Rhode Island developed written materials regarding ACT programs. The Dane County material is in the form of a policy and procedure manual, as well as a whole host of forms used by the clinical teams. Independently, Rhode Island developed a program standards manual that is quite similar to Dane County's policy and procedure manual. It is not a coincidence that they are similar, since both programs were patterned after the original ACT program developed at the Mendota Mental Health Institute by Stein, Test, and Marx. Some material in this book was developed by liberally adapting content from both Dane County's policy and procedure'm anual and Rhode Island's program standards manual; we thank them both for allowing us to do that. In addition, we are especially appreciative to the Mental Health Center of Dane County, Inc., for giving us permission to place, in the appendix of this book, forms used by their ACT clinical teams. These forms will be extremely useful to other ACT teams, especially those in the process of developing.

We are grateful to the National Alliance for the Mentally Ill and to their

Director, Laurie Flynn, for their recognition of the usefulness of the ACT model to help persons with severe and persistent mental illness achieve a stable life of decent quality in the community and to include dissemination of ACT as part of their important anti-stigma campaign.

A special thanks to my wife, Karen Sessler Stein, for her expertise in copyediting and knowledge of grammar. She also showed a remarkable degree of patience and good humor while I (LIS) was deeply immersed in the writing of this book. Many thanks also to Elaine Henry for her administrative assistance to Dr. Santos, to his seven-year-old son, Charlie, and his wife, Barbara, for letting him work when he should have been playing and fixing things, and to his mother, Celida, and in memory of his father, Alberto Sr., for suggesting he attend medical school to supplement his work as a drummer for rock' n' roll bands.

Some of the content of this book was previously published in material authored by Drs. Stein and Santos. We are grateful to the following journal and book publishers for their permission to reprint and/or adapt material previously published by Drs. Stein and Santos: *Health Affairs* of The People to People Health Foundation, Inc., Project Hope for Dr. Stein's paper, "On the Abolishment of the Case Manager" (Fall 1992, 172–177); Praeger Publishers for Dr. Stein's chapter "Persistent and Severe Mental Illness: Its Impact, Status, and Future Challenges," which appeared in R. Schultz and J. Greenley (eds.), *Innovating in Community Mental Health,* an imprint of Greenwood Publishing Group, Inc., Westport, CT; Jossey-Bass, Inc., Publishers, for permission to reprint a portion of Dr. Stein's paper, "Innovating Against the Current," which appeared in *New Directions for Mental Health Services,* no. 56, of which Dr. Stein was the guest editor; American Psychiatric Press, Inc. for material from S. Henggeler and A. Santos (eds.), *Innovative Approaches for Difficult-to-Treat Populations; The American Journal of Psychiatry,* for material from Santos et al.: "Research on Field-based Services: Models for Reform in the Delivery of Mental Health Care to Populations with Complex Clinical Problems," 152(8):1111–1123, 1995, and Santos et al.: "A Community-based Public-academic Liaison Program," *151*(8)1181–1193, 1994; *Psychiatric Services* for material from Burns and Santos: "Assertive Community Treatment: A Research Update," *46*(7):669–675, 1995; Deci et al.: "Dissemination of Assertive Community Treatment Programs," *46*(7)676–678, 1995; Santos et al.: "Providing Assertive Community Treatment for Severely Mentally Ill Patients in a Rural Area," *44*:34-39, 1993; *Community Mental Health Journal* for material in Meisler et al.: "Impact of Assertive Community Treatment on Homeless Persons with Co-occuring

Severe Psychiatric and Substance use Disorders," *33*(2)113–122, 1997; and, finally, to *Administration and Policy in Mental Health* for material which appeared in their special edition on ACT in which Dr. Santos was guest editor (in press). Dr. Santos' work was supported in part by NIMH grants MH46624, MH19466, MH49303, MH53431, MH53558, and MH51852.

Assertive Community Treatment

of Persons with Severe Mental Illness

Introduction

For NAMI families, ACT programs offer security and peace of mind. . . the family for the first time knows that there's going to be a real safety net around their relative, no matter what the problem, no matter what the service need, someone can be reached and someone will respond.

—Laurie Flynn, Director,
National Alliance for the Mentally Ill
from the film, "Hospital Without Walls" (1994)

The goal of services for persons with severe and persistent mental illness is for that person to achieve a stable life of decent quality and to become involved in activities that promote meaningful community living. In the United States, as is true virtually everywhere else, there has been little success in achieving this goal. There are still large numbers of persons who are unnecessarily admitted to hospitals repeatedly and live a poor quality of life between hospitalizations. They may live in isolation or have tenuous interpersonal relationships; they have little to do during the day that they see as useful; they often experience their lives as meaningless and chaotic; and their general health status is often inadequate.

Complicating the problem is the fragmented nonsystem of public mental health care that exists in the United States. Various community and hospital services operate as if the others do not exist; each has its own criteria for admission and rules that clients must follow in order to remain in the program. The services are uncoordinated and non-collaborative, and when clients are denied services, extruded from services, or never apply for them in the first place, no one feels obligated to ensure that their needs are being met. Furthering the problem is the fact that many, if not most, communities do not have all the needed services. In this nonsystem, even when all services are available, a few clients get more than they need, many clients get less than they need, and some get nothing at all. This nonsystem fails service recipients, frustrates families, and undermines the potential effectiveness of the professionals working in it.

The assertive community treatment (ACT) model was designed to provide a solution to this problem. ACT is best conceptualized as a service delivery vehicle or system designed to furnish the latest, most effective and efficient treatments, rehabilitation, and support services conveniently as an integrated package. It serves as the fixed point of responsibility for providing services to a group of individuals with severe and persistent mental illness identified as needing ACT services to achieve any of several desired outcomes (e.g., reduced use of "revolving door" hospital services, increased quality and stability of community living, normalizing activities of daily living such as competitive employment). Services are not time-limited or sequenced. Service intensity varies with changes in desired outcomes. Services are provided for as long as needed, which is usually a matter of years and, for some clients, a lifetime.

The approach is integrative: A multidisciplinary group merges their expertise to provide an array of coordinated services necessary to achieve desired goals. The great majority of the services are provided by the treatment team. However, when other program entities are used, the ACT team remains the fixed point of responsibility, ensuring that the supplemental services are adequate and provided in the context of the whole program.

ACT services are mostly delivered "in vivo," that is, in the community where clients live and work. The team assists to:

- lessen psychoses (duration, intensity, frequency)
- maintain a substance-free lifestyle
- maintain decent and affordable housing in a normative setting
- minimize involvement with law enforcement and criminal justice
- acquire and keep a job
- maintain good general health status
- meet other individual goals

Lessening the duration, intensity, and frequency of psychoses involves close monitoring, rapid stabilization of crises, and ongoing training to enable the client to self-monitor and manage signs and symptoms. Obtaining and retaining decent and affordable housing in a normative setting requires repeated neighborhood interventions. Minimizing involvement with the criminal justice system requires interventions designed to eliminate unlawful activities. It also requires collaborative work with police, the courts, and the jail, so that the ACT program becomes a jail diversion service. Maintaining ideal health status requires ensuring that all health problems are addressed in a timely manner, developing collaborative relationships with primary care providers, and, when necessary, accompanying clients to their appointments. Finally, staff assist clients in meeting other goals as prescribed in their individual treatment plans.

No psychosocial intervention has influenced current community mental health care more than ACT. It has truly revolutionized how we provide services to help people suffering from severe mental illnesses achieve a stable life of decent quality in their community. Further, the model is the most widely researched and validated service system available for the care of this group of disabled individuals. This volume is the first to comprehensively cover the ACT model of community-based care. It gives a brief overview of how persons with severe mental illness have been managed by society over the ages and puts ACT in a historical perspective by describing its development in the early 1970s. It then goes on to explain the treatment approach, from conceptual framework to specific interventions utilized. The book describes in detail the "nuts and bolts" of how the program works on a day-to-day basis and how it involves families and the community at large in a collaborative effort. It provides a set of forms used by an ACT team as templates for documenting client assessments and treatment plans. The book describes how the staff works as a team, makes group decisions, and shares expertise through cross-training. Information is provided as to how the model has been modified for rural settings and for homeless persons and to maximize the opportunity to move persons with severe mental illness into the work force. Information about the model's research base and financing mechanisms are presented in an easy-to-read format.

This book was written to serve a wide audience. It was written so that those interested in operating an ACT program could do so by using this book as a manual; sufficient specific information is presented to start an ACT program from scratch (including necessary paperwork). The book should also be useful to students studying mental illnesses, giving them the opportunity to learn about the nature of suffering from these illnesses and about historical trends in providing services designed to facilitate a stable and meaningful life in the community for individuals with disabling psychiatric disorders.

One final note—how we refer to others has a subtle but powerful effect on what or how we think about them, which, of course, affects how we behave toward them. Throughout this volume, we have made a concerted effort to refer to or about persons with mental illness in a respectful manner. Prejudice against the mentally ill is subtle and widespread. The effect of stigmatization is demoralizing. We all need our consciousness raised, regularly. Thus, for example, we urge readers to join us in not referring to people by their diagnosis. For instance, "Mr. Smith, who is a schizophrenic," should be replaced by, "Mr. Smith, who is a person suffering from schizophrenia." We take this risk in being seen as condescending, because we believe so strongly that society's attitudes towards persons suffering from mental illness must change, and whatever can be done to bring this about, no matter how small it may seem, must be done. If we have failed to be respectful in some instances, we would appreciate it being called to our attention.

Suggested Videotape

Burns, B. J., & Swartz, M. S. (1994). *Hospital without walls.* A videotape presentation on a program for assertive community treatment. Durham, NC: Division of Social and Community Psychiatry, Department of Psychiatry, Duke University Medical Center.

·›»❱❱ 2 ❰❰❰‹·

Stigma and Prejudice

The worst sin towards our fellow creatures is not to hate them, but to be indifferent to them. That's the essence of inhumanity.

—George Bernard Shaw

Human beings have the capacity to identify and empathize with each other. To do so, however, we must get beyond the initial fear (or persistent avoidance) of people who are "different." Only then are we able to appreciate how much alike we really are. It is difficult to dehumanize and treat harshly people whom you know as individuals; that is the major reason why integration is important in neutralizing prejudice.

A major goal of Assertive Community Treatment (ACT) is to help persons with mental disabilities become integrated into their communities as individuals. This goal is unique in the field's history of working with, and relating to, people with mental illness. This chapter provides a brief historical overview of society's relationship to the mentally ill and puts ACT in a historical context.

An unfortunate characteristic of human beings is the tendency to distrust, be suspicious of, and dislike other humans who appear to be different from ourselves. From an evolutionary perspective, this characteristic may have been useful at one time, for example, in keeping other tribes away from your tribe's hunting and gathering territory. However, for the last several thousand years this characteristic has been expressed in all the various prejudices we are familiar with, from racism to religious persecution, resulting in untold miseries for millions of people.

Since the dominant culture varies from place to place, the object of prejudice varies along with it. Hence, racism is evident within the dominant group of most societies. In addition, the objects of prejudice can change over time within the same societies. Spanish Jews, for example, were given a great deal of freedom and tolerance from the middle of the eighth to the four-teenth century, but were severely victimized by rampant prejudice in the fif-teenth century.

In contrast, one group of people has been consistently discriminated against across both time and cultures—those persons who, at times, behave in strange and bizarre ways. In short, persons with mental illnesses have been the most consistently discriminated against group of people in the history of man. The result of that discrimination has varied from, at best, benign neglect, to, at worst, persecution and systematic extermination.

How Mental Illness Was Understood in Ancient Times

In Eastern Mediterranean and North African countries, five-thousand-year-old skulls have been found that showed evidence of trephination. These skulls had openings in them of up to two centimeters in diameter. It is thought that these holes were made by a sharp instrument and that the pro-cedure was performed for therapeutic reasons.

Some of the recipients were believed to be persons who were mentally ill, which at that time, was assumed to be the result of having evil spirits in their heads. The purpose of putting a hole in the head was to allow the evil spirits to be released.

In ancient Greece, persons with severe mental illnesses who behaved strangely were thought to be influenced by angry gods and were undoubtedly abused. Those whose condition was relatively mild were allowed to be free and to roam around but were treated with contempt and humiliation.

Views of the Mentally Ill During the Inquisition in Europe

It is ironic that the renaissance in Western Europe was a particularly dreadful time to be mentally ill. Although notions about what caused people to behave strangely did not change very much, the evil power attributed to the mental-ly ill led to horrendous ways of dealing with them. In 1484, Pope Innocent VIII issued a papal bull in which he essentially stated that those who behaved strangely did so because they were possessed by the devil. Further, he declared that these possessed witches and sorcerers were responsible for vir-tually all the calamities that befell mankind, from crop failure to women being unable to conceive. Two Dominican brothers, Johann Sprenger and Heinrich Kraemer, wrote a three-volume treatise, published within a few years of the Pope's bull, entitled the *Malleus Maleficarum*—the witches hammer. These volumes became the "textbook" of the Inquisition. The first volume made the case that persons who behaved in particularly strange ways did so because they were possessed by the devil. They further stated that people who did not believe this to be true were either ignorant and needed to be educated or showed by their disbelief that they themselves were possessed. The second volume contained very detailed descriptions of behaviors that would indicate that the person displaying them was possessed. Some of these descriptions were so detailed they could be used today to diagnose specific mental disorders. The third volume described how the inquisitor should attempt to free the afflicted person from demonic possession. This initially involved getting the afflicted person to admit to being possessed and to recant. If simply asking the individual to do so failed, there were a series of increasing tortures to convince the person to do so. This was all done with the intent of helping the possessed individual liberate his or her soul and escape eternal damnation. If all tortures failed, then the soul needed to be freed by destroying the body inhabited by the devil. This was ordinarily done by burning at the stake, hanging, or decapitation. The *Malleus Maleficarum* went through nineteen editions over the next few centuries. Over the three hundred years that it influenced the Inquisition, these volumes, and those who practiced its writings, were responsible for the deaths of hundreds of thousands of innocent, mentally ill persons. The last person to die at the hands of the Inquisition was a "witch" who was decapitated in Switzerland in 1782.

Changing Treatment in the Age of Enlightenment

As the Age of Enlightenment began to take hold in Europe and the inquisitors were losing their power, the development of institutions to house society's deviants was well underway. These structures housed the petty criminal, the debtor and the demented, as well as the mentally ill. The conditions for the inmates were quite deplorable, with people chained to walls and even kept in cages.

Two contemporaries, one in England and one in France, led us away from the barbaric treatment of the mentally ill as described above, by beginning the movement to reform these institutions into places that treated their charges with respect and decency. In the late eighteenth century, Philippe Pinel, a French physician, and William Tuke, an English layman, believed that those who behaved in strange and unexplainable ways were doing so because they were mentally ill.

Pinel reformed the Bicêtre and Salpêtrière Hospitals in France by unchaining the inmates and relating to them as reasonable people, treating them with respect, and providing decent conditions. Tuke founded the York Retreat in England and was guided by humanistic ideals and the Protestant ethic. Mentally ill persons at the York Retreat were related to in a respectful manner, were expected to work to the extent they could, and were provided with decent living conditions. The approach William Tuke developed became known as "moral treatment." The number of hospitals utilizing that approach began to increase.

Treatment of the Mentally Ill in America from Colonial Times to 1970

In the American Colonies, the ways in which mental illness was conceptualized and dealt with were heavily influenced by what was going on in Europe. Thus, the Colonies had their witch trials and the execution of innocent people. However, since the Colonies were sparsely populated (compared to Europe), the mentally ill were fortunate to be spared being incarcerated in large institutions where the inmates were treated as animals (sadly, this was to come later, as will be described).

The Colonies did borrow from the English and developed a number of small (less than 200 beds) hospitals that patterned themselves after the York Retreat and gave their patients the benefit of moral treatment. These hospitals were usually affiliated with one of the religious orders and the patients were generally very similar to the staff regarding national origin, religion, and ethnic background.

These hospitals, however, were not available to the masses of eastern and southern Europeans who emigrated to the United States in great numbers in the nineteenth century. These immigrants, often of different religions and certainly of different cultures from the original colonists, did not have moral hospitals to treat their mental illnesses. They were, instead, often kept locked in a room in their home, cared for by their family, or they roamed around being objects of derision by the citizenry. Many ended up in alms houses and incarcerated in jails with common criminals.

Dorothea Lynde Dix, a retired school teacher, was so moved by the plight of those mentally ill who were abused by society that she embarked on a personal crusade. Virtually single-handedly, she advocated that government establish moral treatment hospitals for the indigent mentally ill. She traveled throughout the United States, going from one state legislature to another, pressuring politicians, bureaucrats, citizens, and anyone else who would listen to build government supported hospitals that would provide moral treatment to those who needed it.

She was quite successful, and state after state built hospitals for the mentally ill. Initially, the hospitals functioned just as she envisioned. The patient-to-staff ratio was sufficient to provide moral treatment. The patient populations of the hospitals were small enough to provide decent living conditions. Unfortunately, the number of admissions far exceeded the number of discharges and wards that were initially designed to accommodate twenty-five patients were soon crowded with several times that number. The number of patients per staff member spiraled upwards. This was due, in part, to greater and greater numbers of persons immigrating to the United States, leading to higher admission rates and, in part, to the inability of the staff to therapeutically help patients so that they were well enough for discharge. Mentally ill persons would routinely be admitted to the hospital and spend the rest of their lives there. The hospitals were like isolated fiefdoms where patient labor was used to do much of the work. Since patients worked on the hospital's farm, and in the kitchen and laundry, the cost of keeping a patient in a state hospital was often not more than a few dollars a day. The unclaimed dead were buried in a cemetery on the grounds.

By the 1950s, there were over one-half million Americans living in crowded institutions, receiving little more than custodial care. The conditions in the institutions were deplorable and the general public was either ignorant or disinterested in the plight of the mentally ill living in those institutions. This shameful and unconscionable situation was supported by the eugenics movement, which believed human evolution would be retarded if the mentally ill were permitted to live in society and procreate.

These deplorable conditions were finally brought to public attention through newspaper exposés and films such as *The Snake Pit.* Eventually, the public became aware of the plight of the mentally ill in the state hospitals and efforts to bring about change began to happen. In the United States, the 1960s was the era of liberation and the plight of the mentally ill became a cause consistent with the times. The community mental health movement was, in large part, an attempt to find a solution to the hospital problem described above.

Court cases to ensure the rights of the mentally ill to treatment and due process of law were brought by public interest attorneys. Also, due in part to these legal actions, hospitals were mandated to have greater numbers of staff, were forbidden to exploit patients for labor, and came under public scrutiny regarding conditions for patients within the hospital.

As a result of all these changes, the cost of state hospital care increased manyfold, and the state hospital became a major economic burden on state budgets. In 1965, a new federal program to pay for the medical care of the poor and disabled was enacted into law. The program, called Medicaid, gave states an opportunity to replace state dollars with federal dollars in caring for the state's mentally ill.

One provision of Medicaid was that it did not pay for the hospital costs of mental institutions but would pay for the care of the mentally ill if they were treated in the community. Within the next ten years, the state hospital population in the United States decreased over eighty percent, so that from 1965 to 1975 over 400,000 state hospital patients were discharged from hospitals. Many were transferred to nursing homes, but the great majority were placed in community settings. The movement to the community was facilitated by the availability of antipsychotic medications that were introduced in the early 1950s and in wide use by 1965. However, there is general agreement that the most powerful factor fueling the deinstitutionalization movement to community care was the opportunity for states to shift a large share of the cost from their budgets to the federal government.

The communities, however, were not prepared. In fact, the technology for caring for persons with severe and persistent mental illness in the community had not yet been developed. It was believed that all that was necessary to keep these individuals stable in the community was a place to live and an appointment at the local mental health center, where they could get a prescription for their medication. This turned out not to be the case. There were a number of tragic consequences resulting from our inability to adequately care for severely mentally ill persons in the community:

1. There was a high frequency of relapse back to the psychotic state and, thus, the readmission rate to hospitals increased tremendously.
2. After being readmitted to the hospital and having their psychosis treated, patients were discharged back to inadequate care in the community, only to become psychotic again and start the process all over again. This pattern was so prevalent that it was given the term "revolving door syndrome."
3. Some got lost to care and ended up homeless.
4. Others, found wandering and homeless, committed minor crimes and ended up in the criminal justice system.

This whole state of affairs was tragic for mentally ill persons and their families. There were strong feelings in many sectors of society (mental health professionals, bureaucrats, the public in general) that the deinstitutionalization policy was a great mistake. They believed that everyone, especially the patients, would be better off if the mentally ill lived their lives in hospitals.

By and large, most individuals afflicted with mental illnesses did not agree. Although their lives were difficult in the community, they coveted their autonomy and resisted joining the chorus for massive reinstitutionalization. There were others who resisted, notably, civil rights activists and a small group of mental health professionals who believed that methods could be developed to help the mentally ill live stable and satisfying lives in the community. Interestingly, virtually all of these mental health professionals were persons who had worked in state institutions and fervently believed there had to be a better answer. They were well acquainted with how a total institution restricts life even when it provides a decent environment and empathic care.

The most powerful force preventing a public policy shift back to institutionalism as the primary mode for dealing with the severely mentally ill was the high cost of hospital care. States simply could not afford to do it.

Thus, the opportunity to develop a technology of community care became a possibility, if not a necessity. The first efforts utilized a transitional strategy based on the notion that the mentally ill person needed to move gradually from the hospital to full community living. The initial attempt at this was the halfway-house model, which provided for housing and staff availability twenty-four hours a day on the premises. There was a fixed time limit, usually three to six months, by which time the patients had to move on to a more independent living situation. They were encouraged to get involved in community day programs, such as sheltered workshops, and to receive their psychiatric care at the local mental health center. They were also expected to participate in the running of the halfway house, such as helping with the cooking and cleaning, as a way to learn the skills necessary to live more independently. Some were able to successfully move from halfway houses to more independent living; however, many quickly relapsed and required rehospitalization shortly after leaving the halfway house.

Another model was the day hospital or partial hospital. This model operated just like hospitals in terms of programming and staffing during the day. Patients lived elsewhere and came to the day hospital for treatment. This model was used as an alternative to hospitalization and as a means of reducing length of stay by discharging patients earlier than would be possible if this alternative were not available. Like the halfway house, the day hospital was time limited and conceptualized as a transitional strategy. Also like the halfway house, it was of little assistance to people once they were discharged; consequently, those discharged from partial hospitals experienced high relapse rates.

The Fairweather Lodge was a model developed by George Fairweather, who was dissatisfied with the outcome of patients being discharged from the Veterans Administration hospital in which he worked. The experience there was essentially the same as in the state hospital—a high rate of relapse and rehospitalization. He took groups of long-stay patients and had them work together in the hospital until groups could be formed that got along well together. He then moved a group out into a house in the community where they would live and care for each other. In addition, the group would develop a business, such as providing janitorial services to office buildings, as a means of generating money to help support themselves. Initially, staff would be assigned to the house to help with the process and then would be gradually withdrawn. The model was quite successful but somewhat cumbersome, in that it required starting out with hospitalized patients who were together in the hospital long enough to develop into compatible groups and then move out en masse, live together, work together, and be reliable enough to develop a stable community. It also did not work well for those patients who could not tolerate living in a group situation. The model was, however, an important milestone in recognizing the need for patients to have long-term support of everyday needs in order to live stable lives in the community.

The academic community played a negative role with regard to the state of affairs in America for persons with severe and persistent mental illnesses. Let us remind ourselves, and inform newcomers to our mental health professions, of our misguided accusations that family members in some way had caused their children's illnesses. For readers not familiar with our field's "black eye" with regard to the families of individuals with schizophrenia, a historical note is in order: In the 1950s, a group of influential American academic family therapists formulated the erroneous premise that families caused schizophrenia in their children by repeatedly placing them in psychological "double bind" situations that could be improved through their family-therapy-based treatment strategy. Their work was totally anecdotal and without any empirical validation, yet their theories were widely popularized and readily accepted by professional training programs, who passed this misinformation on to a generation of clinicians from all the mental health disciplines. With time, their treatment efforts were discredited, but by then a lot of harm had been done. Many professionals were left confused and poorly trained. Family members, individually and as a group, very much resented the notion that they had caused their relative's illness. As a result, the relationship between family advocacy organizations and mental health professionals became strained, with residual bad feelings still very much alive today.

Suggested Readings

Aviram, U. (1990). Care or convenience? On the medical-bureaucratic model of commitment of the mentally ill. *International Journal of Law & Psychiatry, 13,* 163–177.

Mechanic, D. (1987). Correcting misconceptions in mental health policy: Strategies for improved care of the seriously mentally ill. *The Milbank Memorial Quarterly, 65,* 203–229.

Rochefort, D. A. (1993). *From poorhouses to homelessness: Policy analysis and mental health care.* Westport, CT: Auburn House.

Torrey, E. F. (1997). *Out of the shadows, confronting America's mental illness crisis.* New York: Wiley.

Origins of Assertive Community Treatment

Did you ever wonder why many consumers are angry?
The day programs in most towns are silly and boring.
The housing, if there is any at all, is in the most run-
down and dangerous of neighborhoods. The jobs we get
trained for are by and large low wage, dead-end jobs with
no real chance for career development.

—Thomas M. Posey,
NAMI President, 1989

Innovation starts with an idea. What happens to the idea once it is exposed to public scrutiny is greatly influenced by the environment surrounding it. If the idea is congruent with the traditions, philosophy, and practice of the environment in which it was spawned, it will be nurtured, protected, and encouraged to grow and bear fruit. If, on the other hand, the idea is contrary to, or inconsistent with, the traditions of its environment, its life is much more hazardous, its rate of growth slower, and its chances of growing strong enough to bear fruit reduced. This chapter is the story of such an idea–an idea originating in an environment eager to encourage innovation but reluctant to permit the development of an innovation that was contrary to its major mode of practice.

Influence of the Environment on Innovation

Innovation is a product; activities to produce it are expected in organizations that identify that product as one of its goals. Thus, we expect innovation from universities and from the research and development sections of industrial corporations. We do not normally expect it from organizations whose primary—

and often only—responsibility is to provide service. In the early 1960s, Mendota State Hospital in Madison, Wisconsin, was a state mental hospital in the business of serving patients by providing clinical treatment and serving society by protecting it from dangerous patients. Not unlike many of the progressive state hospitals around the country, it had a good staff, a large patient population, and high rates of both discharge and readmission. In addition, it had a small office of research and education, staffed by a single individual.

In the mid 1960s, two events occurred that greatly modified the character of the institution. First, the hospital made a major decision to increase its research activities and enlarge its research department. Thus, in a real sense it declared that, in addition to service, the hospital was now seriously in the business of producing innovation. Second, the hospital hired an innovative new director of research and education. The new director, Dr. Arnold Ludwig, was an energetic, creative researcher who was also a skillful administrator. He was successful in getting the hospital to dedicate an entire ward, with a full complement of staff, to research activities. He formed a special treatment unit (STU), a research unit whose primary purpose was to evaluate various psychosocial techniques for the modification of behavior and the rehabilitation of persons with chronic schizophrenia. In addition to the usual ward staff, he attracted two young and talented clinician/researchers, Arnold Marx, a psychiatrist, and Mary Ann Test, a psychologist, to work with him. Together, they designed and implemented a variety of novel psychosocial treatment techniques within a research design context. It was not accidental that the research was focused on psychosocial approaches; Dr. Ludwig believed that persons with schizophrenia were anything but fragile and helpless. Thus, he believed that psychosocial interventions could influence persons with schizophrenia to change from behaving in ways that kept them in the institution to behaving in a manner that would lead to their discharge from the institution.

Although on occasion staff from other units raised objections to some of the treatment approaches being used on the STU, the administration strongly supported the STU and ran interference for that unit, essentially squelching any attempts to disrupt the STU. This was not surprising, since the institution had, by then, identified itself as providing innovation, along with service, as a major goal. And very importantly, the operation of the STU was consistent with the traditions, philosophy, and operation of the hospital. The innovations were carried out in an inpatient setting; the roles of the various professional and paraprofessional groups working on the STU were the same as those on the service units. In essence, the innovations were going with the current and thus received the support of the institution.

A Change in Focus: Going against the Current

Through the programs of the STU, Ludwig, Marx, and Test demonstrated that a variety of novel psychosocial treatment techniques could have an impact on previously unresponsive patients and could significantly enhance their in-hospital functioning. Even when treatment approaches were unsuccessful, they were important learning experiences that led them to consider alternative treatment techniques. The format and outcome of these treatment research programs, as well as process data and theoretical implications, were carefully documented.

While the major emphasis of the projects was on inpatient treatment, staff also gained experience and expertise that would be helpful in providing patients with community care after discharge from STU. However, it was not an uncommon experience for patients who were discharged in a stable condition to be readmitted to the hospital, within a relatively short period of time, once again psychotic. This revolving-door phenomenon was happening not only on the STU, but also on the acute service units of Mendota State Hospital, reflecting a national trend.

When Ludwig left in 1970 to become chairman of the Department of Psychiatry of the University of Kentucky Medical School, one of the authors (LIS) took over his position as Director of Research and Education, and Marx and Test assumed leadership of the STU. These changes in leadership made possible a marked shift in the direction that future STU programs would take. Ludwig had been primarily interested in learning more about using psychosocial techniques in an inpatient setting, whereas Drs. Marx, Test, and Stein were interested in helping patients sustain their community tenure. It became increasingly clear to them that the crucial variable in producing success after discharge was an intensive and sustained program of support and treatment in the community. They decided to change the focus of research from activities in an inpatient setting designed to prepare patients to live in the community to activities in an outpatient setting designed to help patients make a sustained adjustment to community life.

An important factor influencing this shift of focus from inpatient to outpatient treatment was an orientation to mental illness and patients' civil liberties that Drs. Stein and Marx had developed during their residency training. They both received their training from the Department of Psychiatry of the University of Wisconsin Hospital and Clinics. That department, chaired by Dr. Milton Miller, had a very strong antibiological orientation regarding the etiology of mental illness. Carl Whitaker, M.D., a prominent member of the department, was a family therapist who believed and taught that schizophrenia was caused by pathological parenting (a concept that is now recognized as being erroneous). Jay Haley, a charismatic and renowned therapist, was a frequent visitor to the department and shared the same views as Dr. Whitaker. In concert with those views was the department's strong orientation regarding civil liberties. Dr. Seymour Halleck, a nationally known professor in the department, lectured and wrote about how society used psychiatry as a social control agent. He believed that many people, including many diagnosed with schizophrenia, were not really ill but simply behaved in a deviant manner. Psychiatry, he believed, was often used by society to control people behaving strangely by giving them a diagnosis; this permitted society to discount them and/or put them away in a hospital. Further reinforcing these views were the visits and lectures of Dr. Thomas Szasz, who expounded upon his "myth of mental illness" position; his views were essentially the same as Dr. Halleck's. This was during the the early 1960s, a heady time, when being anti-establishment was becoming very much in vogue. Given this strong antimedical bias, coupled with very strong beliefs that the mentally ill were unjustly incarcerated in mental hospitals, it is not surprising that, upon Dr. Ludwig's departure, Drs. Stein and Marx were primed to do community instead of hospital psychiatry. Dr. Test's internship at the progressive Fort Logan Mental Health Center in Colorado, prepared her to be eager to do community work as well.

Drs. Marx, Test, and Stein obtained a small grant to do a pilot study termed, "The Prevention of Institutionalization Program" (PIP), which resulted in a paper entitled "Extrohospital Management of Severe Mental Illness." Following the pilot project, Dr. Marx moved to California, and Drs. Stein and Test wrote a sizable NIMH grant, which led to their studies of community treatment of persons with mental illness. The conceptual framework supporting the interventions proposed in that grant was developed from experiences in the PIP project, as well as from the views of Professor David Mechanic, a distinguished sociologist who headed up the medical sociology section of the University of Wisconsin Department of Sociology. Professor Mechanic liked having a psychiatrist on the faculty of his graduate seminar; Dr. Halleck served that role, and when he left for North Carolina, Professor Mechanic asked Dr. Stein to take Halleck's place. Professor Mechanic held the belief that persons with severe and persistent mental illness needed to have the necessary resources, skills, and supports in order to achieve a stable life in the community. His views were in concert with the observations made by Drs. Marx, Test, and Stein in the PIP study and helped crystallize, for Drs. Stein and Test, the conceptual framework that became the basis of their proposal submitted to NIMH.

A discussion of the immediate changes in staff functions that occurred in both the pilot study and the larger study follows:

Staff would no longer report to the hospital and work on an inpatient ward. Instead, they would report to work at an old house in downtown Madison, Wisconsin, where they would spend approximately forty-five minutes to an hour making plans for how they would work with patients in vivo in the community. For the rest of the time, most of the staff, particularly nurses and aides, would work with patients in the patients' homes, neighborhoods, places of work, and places of recreation. Only the nurses carried beepers and could be contacted at any time; the aides would be out of contact for hours at a time.

In short, from the hospital's point of view, this innovation differed from prior research, in that its operations were not congruent with the customary traditions, philosophy, and practice of the hospital. Thus, rather than going with the current, it was going against the current. This resulted in a change in how the hospital administration related to the research enterprise. Instead of supporting and nurturing the research effort, as it did when the research was carried out in an inpatient setting, the administration was now erecting barriers. Some examples of the administration's concerns were:

Justification for training time. The staff would now be involved in a very different kind of activity. Rather than traditional inpatient work, which is well defined and circumscribed, the staff would be working in an open system. They would be working with patients in the community—patients who, unlike those in the hospital, did not have to do what they were told; staff would have to negotiate with landlords, take care of the complaints of shopkeepers, and work collaboratively with the police and a whole host of agencies from various levels of government. It became clear that the staff would need to be free of their clinical responsibilities for a period of time in order to be trained. The administration had a problem with this: "How can we justify all that staff time with no service being provided?"

Transportation and liability. The staff would need to be mobile and do quite a bit of traveling around town. Customarily, when the hospital needed to transport patients, it used the state cars it had available to them; however, the state was certainly not going to provide state cars to all staff members. Stein and Test understood this and negotiated with the staff about using their own cars. Administrators were concerned that not enough money had been budgeted for reimbursement of travel expenses and that liability issues would not allow staff to transport patients in their own cars.

"Who will be watching the aides?" As noted above, the staff would be

spending their time moving around the community and the aides would be out of contact for hours at a time. The administration was concerned that the aides might not be working when out of contact. "What's to stop them from going to a movie or going home for a period of time?" they wondered.

"Can you eat lunch and not have it count as your lunch hour?" At times, the staff would be involved in teaching patients how to use the local inexpensive restaurants. It would be quite awkward for a staff person teaching the patient how to order lunch not to eat along with the patient. Stein and Test decided that since the staff member was actually working during lunchtime, that period would not be considered a lunch break. The administration raised an objection, asking how the staff could eat lunch without counting that as a lunch break: "Isn't that giving the staff two lunch breaks?"

The administration was in a bind. The hospital had developed a reputation, through Ludwig and his colleagues, as an organization that, in addition to providing service, had an important product—research—to produce. The administration had actively publicized that fact. Now their innovators wanted to do something that was making them uncomfortable. Their innovators wanted to behave in ways that were not consistent with the traditions, philosophy and operation of the institution.

The administration attempted to deal with this bind by putting up enough barriers to influence the innovators to choose an innovation that would be more consistent with the institution. However, Stein, Test, and Marx were convinced that they were onto something important and were iconoclastic enough to be spurred forward by the barriers, rather than succumbing to them.

The administrators were ambivalent. They wanted research, but not the kind their researchers wanted to do. The researchers, on the other hand, were not at all ambivalent. They were committed to doing the research that they had in mind. Through the researchers' persistence, negotiation efforts, and good will, the administration finally okayed a period of time for staff training and allocated money for the needed transportation. The administration was reassured that the liability issue could be managed by the insurers of the staff's cars and that staff would be sufficiently supervised. Also, it finally yielded to the notion that a staff person eating lunch while training a patient should not need to count this as a lunch break.

Now that the barriers of the administration had been overcome, the research could proceed. Upon completion of the PIP study, and with NIMH funding for the Training in Community Living (TCL) study, the latter was begun.

Training in Community Living

Training in Community Living was the name given to the original ACT program; the name change took place many months into the experiment when it became clear that the program was doing much more than training and that the staff had to be quite tenacious in their work with clients and the community. In brief, the program was implemented by mental hospital ward staff who were transplanted to the community. Staff coverage was available twenty-four hours a day, seven days a week. Patient programs were individually tailored and were based primarily on an assessment of the patient's coping-skill deficits and requirements for community living. Most treatment took place in vivo—in patients' homes, neighborhoods, and places of work. More specifically, staff members, on the scene in patients' homes and neighborhoods, taught and assisted them in daily living activities such as laundry upkeep, shopping, cooking, restaurant use, grooming, budgeting, and use of transportation.

In addition, patients were given sustained and intensive assistance in finding a job or sheltered workshop placement, and the staff then continued their daily contact with patients and patients' supervisors or employers to help resolve on-the-job problems. Staff guided patients in the constructive use of leisure time and in the development of effective social skills. They also prodded and supported patients to involve themselves in the community's recreational and social activities. They capitalized on patients' strengths rather than focusing only on their pathology. Also, providing support to patients, patients' families, and community members was a key function of the staff. The program was "assertive"; if a patient did not show up for work, a staff member immediately went to the patient's home to help with any difficulty that might be causing the problem. Each patient's medical status was carefully monitored and treated; medication was routinely used for persons with schizophrenia and manic-depressive disorders.

The innovators of the Training in Community Living (TCL) program recognized that there would be resistance to the dissemination of their program because it ran counter to usual practice; therefore, they gave considerable thought to the barriers that needed to be overcome in order for dissemination to have a chance. They anticipated three barriers.

Barrier 1. Lack of Research Evidence

They were aware that a simple description of the TCL program, with anecdotes of its success, would be easily discounted. Thus, it was determined that a tight research design would be necessary to evaluate the effectiveness of the program. To accomplish this, the TCL model was rigorously evaluated, utilizing a random-assigned controlled experiment.

Further details of the study follow.

All patients seeking admission to the state hospital for inpatient care were screened to see if they met the following three criteria:

1. They had to be residents of Dane County, Wisconsin (Madison and the surrounding area—the county in which the hospital was located).
2. They were required to be between the ages of eighteen and sixty-two years.
3. They could have any diagnosis other than severe organic brain syndrome or primary alcoholism.

Patients meeting these criteria became subjects of the study and were randomly assigned to either the experimental or control group by the admission office staff. Control subjects were treated in the hospital for as long as necessary and then linked with appropriate community agencies. Experimental subjects did not enter the hospital, except in rare instances; instead, they were assigned to the TCL approach for fourteen months, after which they received no further input from the experimental unit staff. The last few months of the fourteen-month period were used to gradually wean the patients, integrating them into existing programs, which were essentially the same programs that treated the control group. Assessment data on all patients were gathered at the baseline (time of admission into the study) and every four months for twenty-eight months, through face-to-face interviews by research staff that operated independently of both clinical teams. Data were reported on experimental subjects who were hospitalized. No patients were excluded on the basis of severity of symptomatology or for any reason other than failure to meet the three specific admission criteria.

A variety of assessment instruments was used, including a form collecting standard demographic data on life situation and economic variables, a measure of symptomatology, and a measure of community adjustment that recorded the patient's living situation, time spent in institutions, employment record, leisure-time activities, social relationships, quality of environment, and subjective satisfaction with life.

Barrier 2. Lack of Cost Data

Drs. Stein and Test were hopeful that their results would show a significant benefit for patients in terms of their tenure in the community and their functioning while in the community. However, they correctly anticipated that they would be questioned about the cost of this treatment as compared to traditional treatment. They were correct in this assumption. Indeed, the scenario that they envisioned happened over and over again: They would present their findings showing a positive clinical outcome and, inevitably, among the first questions asked after the presentation would be the following: "It all sounds well and good, but aren't the costs prohibitive?" They needed to know the answer to that question. Fortunately, a close friend of Dr. Stein's, Professor Burton Weisbrod, was an economist with a national reputation for his work in health economics.

Professor Weisbrod and Dr. Stein were in the habit of sailing Dr. Stein's boat every Sunday morning, and Professor Weisbrod was becoming "hooked" on sailing. Dr. Stein, unabashedly, took advantage of that situation and pressed him to cooperate with himself and Dr. Test in heading up a team to do a benefit-cost study of the TCL model as compared to traditional treatments. Dr. Stein had envisioned it as an "accounting" job and was delighted when Professor Weisbrod turned it into a sophisticated study that took into consideration not only monetary factors but also factors that could not be monetized. This study still stands today as a model for cost-benefit studies of this nature.

Barrier 3. Lack of Data on Family and Community Burden

At the time of the TCL experiment, deinstitutionalization was in full swing. Tens of thousands of patients were being discharged into communities unprepared for their care. In fact, they could not be prepared, because the state of knowledge was such that we really did not know what they needed. We made the incorrect assumption that all patients would need would be periodic visits to the mental health center to get their medication evaluated and represcribed. As a result, their care in the community was grossly inadequate—patients were having a difficult time in the community, relapsing into psychosis and requiring frequent readmissions, being neglected, and ending up homeless or in jail. In fact, the TCL program was designed to address these problems. However, it was not only the patients who were suffering but also family and community members. Much concern was being expressed over the possible burden being placed on family and community members by programs that emphasized community treatment of severely disturbed patients. This viewpoint was being reflected in the literature, which revealed a fear that, although deinstitutionalization might be helpful to patients, it could cause considerable psychological and social disturbance among community members coming into contact with them.

Stein and Test pictured another scenario. If, as they had anticipated, their research showed a positive clinical outcome, and if a benefit-cost study demonstrated that the program would not be economically prohibitive, they could imagine someone saying, in a question-and-answer period, "It sounds fine for the patients, and the costs seem okay, but what about the burden being imposed on family and community members?" To answer that question, they conducted a concurrent third study, designed to measure the social costs of the TCL program as compared with the traditional approach of using short-term hospitalization plus aftercare. Six objective measures and one subjective measure of the burden placed upon the family members of patients in both groups were obtained. Community burden was also assessed through police records of frequency of patient arrests, number of suicidal gestures that required medical attention, and frequency of emergency room use.

Another Potential Barrier:
The Period of Jeopardy—One Tragedy and It Is All Over!

The subjects for the study were patients coming to the state hospital for admission. This was the last stop for patients. The state hospital received patients brought in, handcuffed, by police; patients transferred from psychiatric units of general hospitals because they could not be "managed on that unit"; patients committed by a judge for treatment in a hospital (Stein and Test had an agreement with the judge that if a patient was randomly assigned to the study, they could walk the patient out of the hospital and treat him or her in the community); and patients brought in by family members with a letter signed by a physician that the patient required hospital treatment. Drs. Stein and Test, of course, tried to use good clinical judgment and to hospitalize anyone they thought was imminently suicidal or homicidal (those hospital days would show up in the results as charged against experimental patients), but they were interested in "pushing the limits" and trying to find out if they could treat virtually all potential admissions who were not suicidal or homicidal. Thus, it was necessary for the vast majority of patients to be treated in the community rather than being admitted to the hospital. This meant they had to do a balancing act: if they were too cautious, the experiment would lose a great deal of meaning and impact, but if they were not cautious enough, serious harm could be done.

As it turned out, the experimental group only hospitalized twelve of sixty-five patients for a mean of eleven days per patient; thus, a great many highly symptomatic patients were not admitted but were treated in the community. However, the program was in constant jeopardy. If, within the first few months, they had one tragedy—a suicide, a homicide, a rape, or some other behavior that would bring the program notoriously to the public's attention—it would have been all over. One tragedy, and they would get a call from the hospital superintendent telling them to close up shop and come home. *This sort of jeopardy is rarely true of innovative programs that do not run contrary to the current.* For example, early in the game of renal transplantation the mortality rate was extremely high in terms of the short amount of time patients lived following the transplant. However, no one stopped the transplant program, even though dialysis had been perfected sufficiently to keep patients alive for long periods of time. Running against the current is hazardous business, and Stein and Test were extremely fortunate in not having had a tragedy that would have prematurely shortened the life of their program.

Briefly, the results of the experiments are as follows: The research was designed to have two phases of clinical intervention for the experimental group. The first phase was twelve months of intensive involvement in TCL, followed by two months of weaning the patient onto the existing system; in the second fourteen-month phase, experimental patients received, in essence, the same clinical intervention as the control group. The results of the first fourteen months showed a striking advantage for experimental patients over control patients. Of the sixty-five patients in the control group, fifty-seven were hospitalized for a mean of thirty-six days per patient. In addition, the control patients experienced a 60 percent readmission rate, which was approximately what they had been experiencing prior to coming into the study, and which was the common percentage of readmissions reported nationally by public mental hospitals. In the experimental group, on the other hand, only twelve of sixty-five patients were hospitalized, for a mean of eleven days. Of great importance was the fact that the revolving door was virtually eliminated, with a readmission rate under 10 percent.

Other significant differences favoring the experimental group over the control group are as follows: symptomatology, employment, social relationships, and, very importantly, subjective satisfaction with life. There was no measure in which the control group did better than the experimental group.

In the second fourteen-month period, when the experimental group was being treated with conventional treatment, the gains made during the first period began to deteriorate. There was a gradual, but definite, increase in hospital use by the experimental group, moving toward the rehospitalization rate of the control group. Likewise, the improved social relationships decreased, subjective satisfaction with life decreased, symptomatology increased, and time spent in sheltered employment began to decline sharply. The only gain made by the experimental group in the first phase that did not deteriorate was money earned in competitive employment.

At first blush, this deterioration in the second phase was a disappointment for Stein and Test. However, on further consideration, they came to see this finding as the most important one of the study. Specifically, it clearly demonstrated that the most common strategy being used in mental health to date was failing the patients. That strategy was a time-limited design: Day treatment programs were set up for six months or one year, after which time it was expected that the patient would no longer need them; supportive psychotherapy was set up for a specific period, after which time patients were no longer to need it; living situations were structured to be transitional in nature, whereby it was expected that, after a specified period, the patient would have to move on to a permanent living situation. All of these strategies were based on a "cure" or "preparation" model. What this experiment made clear was that the field needed to shift from a time-limited model to a model that provided services indefinitely. In retrospect, it seems obvious that when one deals with an illness that one does not know how to prevent or cure—and that is, therefore, chronic in nature—the intervention, likewise, must be long-term in nature.

Another important finding of the study was that patients needed a wide range of help in making a sustained and satisfactory life in the community. Thus, treatment programs needed to expand their interest from just psychological interventions to interventions that addressed such everyday problems as material resources (food, shelter, clothing, and medical care). In addition, staff needed to add some of the following to their repertoire of "helping" functions: teaching coping skills to meet the demands of community life; providing enough support to keep the patient motivated to persevere and remain involved with life; helping families and patients work through their problems utilizing a problem-solving approach rather than a psychotherapeutic approach; and supporting and educating community members who were involved with patients—such as law enforcement personnel, agency people, landlords, shopkeepers, and so on—to help them relate in a manner both beneficial to the patients and acceptable to the community members. Finally, these interventions needed to be carried out by a team of workers that assertively worked in vivo when necessary, helping patients and the community with the above.

A benefit-cost analysis should be seen not as a mechanism for deciding mechanically on the allocation of funds and resources among programs, but as a structure for weighing advantages and disadvantages (that is, for organizing knowledge). Considering all the forms of benefits and costs that were derived in monetary terms, the experimental program cost more but provided additional benefits, compared with conventional treatment. However, the added benefits—some $1,200 per patient per year—were nearly $400 more per patient per year than the additional costs. Also, a number of the benefits and costs measured in quantitative but nonmonetary terms showed additional advantages of the community-based experimental program (decrease of symptomatology, increased satisfaction with life, and so on). The bottom line of the economic study was that the differences in costs between the experimental program and the control program were small, whereas the benefits, especially the clinical benefits, were dramatically greater for the experimental group.

As noted earlier, much concern had been raised over the possible burden placed on family and community members by programs that emphasize community treatment of severely disturbed patients. In sum, all measures showed that the TCL program resulted in no more burden on the family or community than the traditional approach. The large amount of support provided to patients, families, and community members in the experimental approach was probably responsible for there being no increase in burden despite the fact that severely disturbed patients were treated in the community.

The major consequence of this innovation in the treatment arena was to change how we think about treating persons with severe and persistent mental illness. The principles of having no arbitrary time limits for programs and broadening mental health intervention to include helping patients with housing, finances, shopping, food preparation, laundry, and so on are now well accepted. It is also now well accepted that treatment must not be facility-bound, whether that facility be a hospital or a mental health center, and that staff must work in the field with the patient. When Stein and Test first advocated those principles, they met with a great deal of resistance, couched primarily in terms suggesting that those functions are not mental health functions. There have also been a variety of consequences for patients, staff, and the community.

Consequences for patients must be seen in context. Virtually all communities in the United States now say they're providing community support services. However, where those services do not follow the principles outlined in this book or where they are so inadequately provided as to have little impact on patients, there are serious negative consequences for patients: a high relapse rate, homelessness, and a drift into the criminal justice system. On the other hand, several studies have shown that when a well functioning ACT program is available to patients, they do very well.

Over the past fifteen years, there has been an interesting shift in how patients have learned to cope with stress. When the primary mode of treatment for persons with severe and persistent mental illness was the hospital, patients learned to use the hospital as a major coping mechanism. Working with patients who use this coping mechanism is very different from working with patients who have learned to take advantage of the supportive system available to them in the community. Specifically, it has taken a great deal of effort to keep that earlier group of patients out of the hospital long enough— and to see them through enough episodes of stress—for them to learn to use the community system. Patients who have had access to a good community system from early on in their illness have never learned to use the hospital as a coping mechanism and, subsequently, are much easier to work with.

Turnover on well functioning ACT teams is very low. When queried, staff often give the following types of responses:

- The work is very professionally satisfying, staff get a lot of responsibility and autonomy, and the results of what you do are very apparent.
- The work is very personally satisfying for primarily two reasons, you get to know clients very well because you work with them on a daily basis over a long period of time, and it is personally gratifying to see persons you have come to care for make so much progress.
- Working within a team structure makes it all possible and gives the support and camaraderie that is absolutely essential in doing this kind of work.

Many ACT teams from around the country have a number of staff who, like the original ACT team, spent many years working in hospitals. They all say they could not go back to hospital work. In the hospital they were all told that they were important members of the team, but, in fact, they felt that not much attention was paid to what they had to say. At staff meetings, the psychiatrist spoke, then the psychologist, and not much time or interest was given to what other members of the team thought. The situation on the ACT team was very different; staff spent most of their time working independently in the community with clients. At the daily staff meetings, when a staff member spoke, everyone listened intently, because that staff member knew, better than anyone else, the person under discussion. In the hospital, staff experienced their job as "carrying out orders." On the ACT team they were important in the decision-making process and while out in the field they frequently made important decisions on the spot. It is little wonder, then, that they much preferred working on an egalitarian team in the community rather than a hierarchical one in the hospital. Another, very important factor reported by former hospital employees was that in the hospital all they saw were the system's failures—the same people coming back all the time. On the ACT team, they saw their successes.

The effect on the community was very interesting. Since the programs were providing a great deal of support to patients and to their families, they received a lot of support from families in return. Landlords, on the whole, were not unhappy with having a large number of chronic mentally ill people living in the community, since it increased the number of available renters. They were provided with a staff that was available to them twenty-four hours a day if problems arose; even more important, the staff ensured that the rent was paid on time.

The business community, on the whole, was unhappy with the situation. They had people who appeared eccentric coming into their stores and often spending a lot of time there. The staff was always available to shopkeepers, but what the shopkeepers really wanted was for the staff to keep patients out of their stores. The staff, having a strong commitment to patients' rights did not, of course, do that. Instead, staff worked closely with the shopkeepers, modeling for them how they should relate to patients and, in addition, giving them tactful lectures about how, in a free society it is necessary to tolerate deviant behavior as long as that deviant behavior is not law-breaking.

There were several episodes where staff had to threaten to go to court if patients' civil rights were not honored. For example, the local YMCA was often used to house patients for short periods of time until permanent housing could be found for them. Local businessmen, who used the YMCA during the day for their exercise workouts, began to complain about the mentally ill persons they would run into in the lobby. The Board of Directors of the YMCA met and attempted to resolve the problem by making a rule that anyone with a psychiatric history could not utilize YMCA housing. Staff met with the board and had to threaten a court action if they did not rescind that policy. They eventually rescinded it and, in fact, became active in providing support to the mentally ill persons using their facility, not only by supporting them in the YMCA lobby but by starting a club for them in the community as well.

Not all stories end so happily. Throughout the United States, downtown businesses with insufficient parking have lost business to suburban shopping centers. This has also been the case in Madison. At one point, the downtown business people decided that the increasing visibility of mentally ill persons in the downtown area was the cause of their business decline. There were headlines in newspapers stating this as a major problem for downtown business. In fact, a city council member attempted to pass a resolution in the City Council to have buses pick up mentally ill persons and drop them off at the suburban shopping centers. This resolution, of course, did not pass, but it was a reflection of feelings that people had.

Now, some years later, this is no longer an issue. The community, on the whole, is not happy about the situation, but they have come to accept the fact that many persons with severe and persistent mental illness are living among them. They are aware that mental health professionals are available around the clock to come and help when necessary and, most important, they are aware that they cannot do anything about "getting rid of these people." Indeed, the community seems to have accepted the fact that persons with serious and persistent mental illness are now a permanent fixture. This change has taken at least a decade.

Suggested Readings

Marx, A. J., Test, M. A., Stein, L. I. (1973). Extrohospital management of severe mental illness. *Archives of General Psychiatry, 29,* 505–511.

Meisler N., & Santos, A. B. (1997). From the hospital to the community: The great American paradigm shift. In S. W. Henggeler & A. B. Santos (Eds.), *Innovative approaches for difficult-to-treat populations.* Washington, DC: American Psychiatric Press.

Stein, L. I., & Test, M. A. (1980). Alternative to mental hospital treatment. I: Conceptual model, treatment program, and clinical evaluation. *Archives of General Psychiatry, 37,* 392–397.

Test, M. A., & Stein, L. I. (1980). Alternative to mental hospital treatment. III: Social cost. *Archives of General Psychiatry, 37,* 409–412.

Weisbrod, B. A., Test, M. A., & Stein, L. I. (1980). Alternative to mental hospital treatment. II: Economic benefit-cost analysis. *Archives of General Psychiatry, 37,* 400–405.

4

ACT Research and Dissemination

Rigorous empirical evaluation of all current mental health and substance abuse treatments and services, demonstrating clinical and cost-effectiveness, is essential to ensure that services provided are indeed beneficial. Policymakers should make use of such information when making decisions regarding funding priorities. This information should lead policymakers to design systems of care mixing effective programs, that is, programs known to produce specifically desired outcomes with certain populations.

Research on ACT services has been a hallmark of ACT program development, as well as a truly unique phenomenon in our field. Never before has a clinical service delivery system been so carefully scrutinized: ACT is the most empirically studied of all community mental health program approaches in existence today (see Table 4-1).

Since the seminal studies in Madison in the 1970s, there have been over a dozen randomized clinical trials in the United States, Australia, Great Britain, and Canada. This body of research provides strong evidence of overall effectiveness for the service system. The first two Madison-based ACT demonstrations set the gold standard for the many replications that followed. Subsequent studies utilized many aspects of the Madison studies: the operational elements of the intervention to be used in subsequent studies; the research instrument's measurement domains (symptoms, hospitalizations, living status, role functioning, quality of life, and overall economic costs); and the research design–randomized clinical trials, allowing a comparison of outcomes with those of a community's standard "hospital and aftercare" services.

The specific benefits of ACT that are variously demonstrated in this large body of work include (see Table 4-1):

- Increased stability of mental status and time out of hospitals.
- Reduced hospital costs.

TABLE 4-1
CONTROLLED RESEARCH ON ACT

Year	Site	Investigators	Illness Phase*	Clinical and Psychosocial Outcomes
1973	Madison, Wisconsin	Marx, Test & Stein	Unstable	ACT more effective (5 mo. trial) in reducing use of hospitals and ER's, in improving residential status, and in preserving occupational status
1980	Madison, Wisconsin	Stein,Test & Weisbrod	Unstable	ACT more effective (12 mo. trial) in reducing use of hospitals, nursing homes, and law enforcement services; in improving residential status, socialization, instrumental functioning, and symptom profiles
1983	Sidney, Australia	Hoult & Reynolds	Unstable	ACT more effective (12 mo. trial) in reducing use of hospitals and ER's; in improving instrumental functioning, symptom profile, residential status, and occupational activity
1985	Grand Rapids, Michigan	Mobray & Muldar	Stable	ACT more effective (30 mo. trial) in reducing use of hospitals and law enforcement services; and in improving instrumental functioning and residential status
1988	3 sites in Indiana	Bond,Miller, et al.	Stable	ACT more effective (6 mo. trial) in reducing use of hospitals in 2 of 3 sites
1989	Santa Clara, California	Jerrell & Hu	Stable	ACT reduced use of hospitals and ER's. Improvements in functioning and quality of life at 12 mo. not present at 24 mo.
1990	Chicago, Illinois	Bond, Witheridge, Dincin, et al.	Stable	ACT more effective (12 mo. trial) in reducing use of hospitals, and in improving instrumental functioning, satisfaction with life, and residential status
1992	London, England	Marks,Muijen, Conolly,et al.	Unstable	ACT more effective (20 mo. trial) for symptoms, social functioning, patient and family satisfaction, and reduced use of hospitals
1994	London, England	Audini, Marks, Laurence, et al.	Stable	ACT treated subjects in study above randomized into ACT or standard services with only significant difference at 45 mo. being increased family and patient satisfaction
1992	London, England	Merson, Tyrer & Onyett	Unstable	ACT more effective than usual hospital and aftercare (3 mo. trial) regarding symptoms, satisfaction with services, and reducing use of hospitals
1992	Madison, Wisconsin	Test et al.	Stable	ACT more effective (in first 2 of 12 year trial) in reducing use of hospitals and improving residential status
1994	10 VA sites in Northeast	Rosenheck	Stable	ACT more effective in reducing use of hospitals (24 mo. trial)
1992	St. Louis, Missouri	Morse et al.	Mixed	For homeless sample, ACT more effective for satisfaction with program, number of days homeless, and use of community resources
1992	New York, New York	McFarlane et al.	Stable	ACT plus family psychoeducation more effective in reducing use of hospitals and facilitating and maintaining client employment

*Phase of illness at the point of recruitment into the study.

- Improvements in adherence to medication regimens.
- Reduced untoward medication side effects.
- Reduced symptom severity.
- Enhanced residential stability.
- Enhanced role functioning, including employment status.
- Improved overall quality of life.

The most consistent significant finding across studies is the greater stability in community living with reduced use of the hospital. People live more independently without increased burden to families.

In studies that target specific problems (homelessness, substance use, unemployment) there is an emerging trend suggesting that specialized interventions of various intensities and complexities will be necessary to target specific desired outcomes. For example, a powerful effect is seen by merging ACT with family psychoeducation in boosting program effectiveness in reducing rates of illness relapse.

Regarding costs, in the largest ACT study to date, a multi-site Veterans Administration project with random assignment to 10 sites in the northeastern United States, nearly 1,000 frequent users of hospital inpatient facilities were followed for two years after discharge into either an ACT system or to a standard aftercare system. Overall, inpatient status was one-third less in the ACT group. The average total cost (including inpatient and outpatient services) was 20 percent less for the ACT group. Two subgroups demonstrated lowest costs, those over 45 years of age and those with the highest rates of hospitalization. Recipients of ACT services lived more independently and were more satisfied with services.

Note that the use of hospitalization is more likely in communities where other non-hospital crisis intervention strategies are not available. Additionally, hospital utilization may not be comparable in rural vs. urban settings, since grossly psychotic, bizarre, eccentric, or other deviant behaviors are better tolerated in rural than urban settings, where they would more likely result in an intervention.

There are several studies in progress in which the control conditions are community mental health centers that provide comprehensive but less coordinated services, including all ten core elements of the federal Community Support Program systems model (see Table 4-2). These studies may shed light on the effects of incorporating key principles of ACT (e.g., fixed point of accountability for care, assertive outreach, practical assistance, community-based contacts, support to social networks) within larger systems of care that incorporate a variety of programs and case management approaches.

TABLE 4-2
Elements of Community Support Systems (CSS) for Seriously Mentally Ill Adults
and their Compatibility with Assertive Community Treatment (ACT)

CSS Principles*	Compatibility with ACT**
Services should be based on and responsive to the needs of the client rather than the needs of the system or the needs of providers; empower clients and build upon their assets and strengths in order to help them maintain a sense of identity, dignity, and self-esteem; and be racially and culturally appropriate.	ACT services are planned, implemented, and revised in accordance with client's needs, strengths and preferences in a fashion designed to maximize community integration and tenure. The team provides longitudinal care, thus capitalizing on in-depth knowledge of the individual and trust established over the long-term clinical relationships.
Services should be available whenever they are needed and for as long as they are needed; be provided in a variety of ways, with individuals able to move in and out of the system as their needs change; be adapted to meet the special needs of subgroups (substance users, mentally retarded, hearing impairments, the elderly, young adults, youth in transition to adulthood, and persons who are homeless or inappropriately placed within the correctional system).	ACT services are available around the clock, without time limit, are fluid in intensity, and are fully mobile. The ACT system is highly adaptable and has been used effectively with homeless, rural, adolescent, substance abusing, hearing impaired and developmentally disabled clients with severe mental illnesses.
Services should be offered in the least restrictive, most natural setting possible. Clients should use the natural supports in the community and be integrated into the normal living, working, learning, and leisure-time activities of the community.	Clinical and rehabilitative services are community field-based or "in-vivo," that is, in a natural community and neighborhood environment.
Service providers should be accountable to the users and monitored to assure quality of care and continued relevance to client needs. Consumers and families should be involved in planning, implementing, monitoring, and evaluating services.	ACT staff is held accountable for their productivity and their client's outcomes (satisfaction, compliance with treatment, housing arrangements, community tenure,etc.).
Services should be coordinated through agreements that require ongoing communication and linkages between participating agencies and the various levels of government. Coordination must occur at the client, community, and state levels. Mechanisms should be in place to ensure continuity of care and coordination between hospital and community services.	ACT services are "self-contained," with the team serving as a fixed point of responsibility for the care of its client caseload. They are the direct providers of all services and will respond to all needs rather than referring clients for specialized services to other agencies or service units. Performance contracts that attend to desired outcomes will maximize same.
Service components include client identification and outreach; mental health treatments; crisis response services; health and dental care; housing; income support and entitlements; peer support; family and community support; rehabilitation services; protection and advocacy; and case management.	ACT services include clinical assessments and treatments including medication administration and monitoring, crisis services, and long-term clinical relationship; support including assistance with basic needs (housing, etc), social environment, and family relations; and direct assistance with instrumental functioning (work, activities of daily living).

* Adapted from Stroul, B. A. (1989). Community support systems for persons with long-term mental illness: A conceptual network. *Psychosocial Rehabilitation Journal, 12*, 9–26.

** Adapted from Test, M. A. (1992). Training in community living. In R. P. Liberman (Ed.), *Handbook of psychiatric rehabilitation*. New York: Macmillan.

ACT Dissemination

Dissemination of new psychosocial service models is generally uneven. In the United States, hospital-based models appear to disseminate at a faster rate than community-based models. For example, the idea of moral treatment hospitals spread rapidly from the York retreat in England to the colonies in America, and it was not long after Scotland's Maxwell Jones described the "therapeutic community" that it swept through the hospitals in the United States—almost overnight, state hospitals, as well as private hospitals throughout the country, developed programs resembling the "therapeutic community." On the other hand, George Fairweather had a difficult time getting his "Lodge Program" disseminated—largely, in our judgment, because it ran against the current and significantly changed the day-to-day functioning of staff, as well as the power differential between patients and staff.

Fidelity of the model replications are often questionable. For example, one wonders whether Jones would have certified all those "therapeutic communities" in the U.S. as fulfilling his requirements. Although in Jones' "therapeutic community" the roles of staff vis-à-vis one another and the power differential between staff and patients changed, that was rarely the case in the "therapeutic communities" spreading throughout our state hospitals in the United States. In practice, the "therapeutic community" movement remained consistent with the traditions, philosophy, and operation of the mental hospital and was, therefore, nurtured by them.

When the ACT idea was first exposed to public scrutiny, it did not greatly influence the environment surrounding it. The idea was not congruent with the traditions and practice of the mental health sector. In fact, it was directly contrary to usual practices and inconsistent with usual procedures of the health business environment. Its course was hazardous and its survival was tenuous; it was rarely nurtured or protected financially. Its growth was not encouraged by administrators, clinicians, or academicians.

Wide dissemination of this model would have enormous consequences for how and where mental health professionals in the public system would be working. It would mean that the primary locus of care would shift from the hospital to the community, with a concomitant reduction in the numbers of hospitals and the numbers of the employees required to work in them. That would entail a major shift in funding—from hospitals to communities. Thus, it would have an enormous effect on the power base of the administrators in state government who would lose those funds. In addition, it would decrease the power of employee unions, because they are much stronger in hospital settings than in most community settings. Staying with the imagery employed earlier in this book, "innovating against the current," wide dissemination would be akin to swimming against a tidal wave.

Not surprisingly, resistance came from many quarters. Hospitals decried this movement as being harmful to patients and pointed to tragedies that had happened all over the country during the movement of deinstitutionalization. They, of course, neglected to point out that these tragedies were happening where there were inadequate services for patients in the community. In some states, the hospital unions have been so politically powerful as to essentially block effective dissemination of these kinds of programs. Mental health workers doing traditional psychotherapy in the community, who did not want to change what they were doing, were also highly resistant to any new program that would require them to practice differently.

Fortunately, certain forces were exerting pressure to develop the kinds of community programs that would keep mentally ill persons stable in the community and reduce hospital use. State governments were feeling the economic pinch of rising hospital costs and were anxious to reduce those costs. In addition, they could legitimately buttress their argument that they did not need so many beds by pointing to the effectiveness of community programs in helping this population.

When those resistant to change were confronted with the successes of ACT, they were asked how in the world could they continue to resist change in light of the positive patient outcomes. The response they gave was unanticipated and frustrating to counter. They readily admitted that the program was successful in helping patients, that it was economically feasible, and that it did not increase family or community burden; but they quickly pointed out that the program was a "model" program and added, "We all know model programs are developed by especially energetic and creative people and will only work if those kinds of people are running it, and further, that these programs are only specific to the area in which they were developed and have limited usefulness in terms of transportability."

What was so frustrating about trying to fight this barrier was that it was the classic "Catch 22," with the "catch" going something like this: For a program to be even considered for exportation, it must, of course, prove its effectiveness; if it is effective, however, it is then obviously a "model" program, and we all know that model programs have limited usefulness in terms of transportability. To support this argument, proponents generally cited other innovations in health care, from transplant surgery to use of the CAT scan, and pointed out how quickly they had become routine procedures. They argued that the fact that ACT programs had not developed as quickly as other health innovations proved that ACT programs must require very energetic and creative people and a very special, receptive environment, thus limiting the concept's transportability.

In the early years, the argument was constantly being made that for ACT to work it needed very special people and very special places. It was the primary rationalization for why programs like this could not be widely implemented. Now, over two decades later, it is rare to encounter that objection because programs like this are being developed in many areas at an accelerating rate. This argument failed to take into consideration several crucial factors that influence how quickly an innovation becomes standard practice. As an example, kidney transplants and CAT scans were innovations that were consistent with the traditions, philosophy, and practice of their respective fields. Indeed, in those fields, the development of new technology is constantly sought after and quickly disseminated. These innovations do not change the basic practices of the clinicians and, very importantly, do not change the hierarchy or role relationships of the key players. The new innovations are frequently made by medical school faculty and first put into operation in teaching hospitals. Thus, they are quickly incorporated into the curriculum and trainees are motivated to emulate their faculty role models in practicing the innovation when they leave training. Although these innovations are often made by especially energetic and creative people, the practitioners of these innovations do not need to share these characteristics; they need only to be able to competently do the work. Further, the innovation itself supports the established structure and, in return, is supported by it. Given these conditions, it is not surprising that dissemination of practices that do not challenge the status quo occurs rapidly.

Contrast that with the ACT program: Although the innovators, Drs. Stein and Test, eventually joined university faculties, the innovation was done while they worked in a public setting and the program itself was developed in a public setting, not a university. Rather than being consistent with the traditions, philosophy, and practice of the field, the ACT program was incompatible with them. A hundred years of hospital treatment, as the primary locus of care for persons with serious and persistent mental illness, was challenged. The basic practice of clinicians changed dramatically from individual and group psychotherapies in an institutional setting to an approach emphasizing community support and rehabilitation in a community setting. This new model required a change in the role relationships of the key players, from a hierarchical model to a much more egalitarian one. This became necessary since so much of the hands-on work and patient contact was being done by nonmedical mental health professionals and paraprofessionals outside of medically oriented institutions. Because this innovation occurred outside of the universities, students in the professional schools were not being prepared to do this kind of work; on the contrary, they were still being trained to do traditional work and were being taught by their role models, the faculty, who were themselves practicing in the traditional way. In short, the innovation of using the community as the primary locus of care for persons with severe and persistent mental illness was not compatible with the established structure or supported by it; in fact, it was actively resisted by it. Therefore, it is not at all surprising that dissemination of this innovation required much more time.

Given the above conditions, it is really surprising how rapidly the innovation has progressed, and, indeed, how much (in terms of standard practice) things have changed because of ACT. In the 1970s, the notions of staff outreaching to people in their homes and neighborhoods, supporting them in permanent supported living arrangements, and utilizing alternatives to hospitalization when relapse occurred were seen as foreign to mental health practice. These practices are now generally accepted as necessary. In the 1970s, having a team designated to provide community-based continuing care to persons who were resistant to treatment and who were seriously and persistently mentally ill was an innovation that existed only in Madison, Wisconsin.

Now, ACT programs are operating in many communities from coast to coast and proliferating rapidly. They are known by many names, such as Program of Assertive Community Treatment (PACT), Continuous Treatment Teams (CTT), Mobile Community Treatment (MCT), or, as in Wisconsin, Community Support Programs (CSP). In addition to the dissemination throughout Wisconsin, there has been state-wide, closely replicated dissemination in Michigan, Rhode Island, and Delaware. Programs with varying degrees of adherence to the Madison model are operating in many other states (see Table 4-3) and in Canada, Australia, and Great Britain, as well.

The National Alliance for the Mentally Ill (NAMI) is currently supporting the development of ACT programs nationwide because they know ACT is helpful to the population in which they are interested. There are now national conferences on ACT. In the 1970s, none of the schools involved in teaching mental health professionals were training them how to do this kind of work. Now, a growing number of schools are doing so; there are now enough programs in operation to justify broadened dissemination into the curricula of all mental health and substance abuse specialists' professional training programs.

The evident effectiveness of ACT in engaging seriously mentally disabled persons in continuous community care, reducing their utilization of

TABLE 4-3 1995 Estimates of ACT Dissemination in the U.S.*			
STATE	**Number of programs**	**STATE**	**Number of programs**
Alabama	4	Missouri	8
Alaska	2	New Hampshire	10
Arizona	5	North Dakota	6
Arkansas	1	Ohio	5
California	3	Oklahoma	1
Connecticut	6	Oregon	1
Delaware	11	Pennsylvania	3
Florida	4	Rhode Island	6
Idaho	6	South Carolina	6
Illinois	7	Douth Dakota	2
Indiana	7	Tennessee	4
Kentucky	1	Texas	1
Maryland	14	Vermont	9
Massachusetts	2	Virginia	3
Michigan	86	Wisconsin	67
Minnesota	1	Wyoming	3

*Data from Deci, P. A., Santos, A. B., Hiott, D. W. et al. (1995). Dissemination of assertive community treatment programs. *Psychiatric Services, 46,* 676-678.

hospitals, and improving their capacity for independent living is particularly important when public and private sector payers are seeking to limit the growth in health care expenditures. The recent trend of rapid dissemination of ACT approaches, nationally, is likely to continue and accelerate.

If policymakers understand that it is no more expensive to provide quality treatment in the community and that mentally ill persons and families are more satisfied, it may then become possible to shift the financial incentive from hospital-based to community care. At such a time, academic institutions will, of necessity, change their principal training focus from a team-oriented institutional approach to a team-oriented approach in the community.

Finally, when thinking about the problems inherent in innovation and dissemination, we must take into account two factors that have not received sufficient attention. First and most important, the degree to which the innovation challenges the traditions, philosophy, and thus practice of the field in which the innovation is taking place must be considered. The more an innovation runs against the current, the more obstacles it will have to overcome before being supported and disseminated. Second, when thinking about dissemination of health care models that challenge traditional practice, the time frame we adopt must be different from those we use for health care models congruent with the established structure. Regarding innovations running against the current, we must think in terms of decades rather than months or years. Keeping these two factors in mind can help smooth the process of innovation.

Suggested Readings

Burns, B. J., & Santos, A. B. (1995). Assertive community treatment: An update of randomized trials. *Psychiatric Services, 46,* 669–675.

Deci, P. A., Santos, A. B., Hiott, D. W., et al. (1995). Dissemination of assertive community treatment programs. *Psychiatric Services, 46,* 676–678.

Olfson, M. (1990). Assertive community treatment: An evaluation of the experimental evidence. *Hospital and Community Psychiatry, 41,* 634–641.

Rosenheck, R., Neale, M., Leaf, P., et al. (1995). A multi-site experimental cost study of intensive psychiatric community care. *Schizophrenia Bulletin, 21*(1), 129–140.

Taube, C. A., Morlock, L., Burns, B. J., & Santos, A. B. (1990). New directions in research on assertive community treatment. *Hospital and Community Psychiatry, 41,* 642–647.

Test, M. A. (1992). Training in community living. In R. P. Liberman (Ed.), *Handbook of psychiatric rehabilitation.* New York: Macmillan.

Characteristics of the Clinical Population

The basic goal of helping people to live a stable life of decent quality in a meaningful environment requires an understanding of the targeted population. Severe and persistent mental illnesses (i.e., schizophrenia, schizoaffective and bipolar disorders) are among many medical illnesses that are, by the nature of their course, chronic conditions. There are large numbers of disorders for which we know no cure, but about which we know enough to minimize disability and improve daily functioning. In fact, in the United States, physicians spend most of their time providing care to persons suffering from incurable diseases such as diabetes, hypertension, coronary artery disease, asthma, arthritic conditions, etc.

Each of these has an "out-of-control" and a "stable" phase. For example, the out-of-control phase of diabetes is diabetic coma; for coronary artery disease, it is severe chest pain; for the arthritic diseases it is swollen and painful joints. Clinical interventions are directed towards reducing the frequency, severity, and duration of the out-of-control phase of the illness and increasing the duration of the stable phase. During the stable phase, the person continues to require care because the disease manifests its long-term impairments. For example, the long-term impairments in arthritis are a limitation in joint movement and a low level of pain; for coronary artery disease, it is a limitation of vigorous activity. During the stable phase, treatment focuses on reducing disability and improving functioning. It is of paramount importance to recognize that the frequency, severity and duration of the out-of-control phase is directly related to the quality of the care received during the stable phase. The better the care during the baseline stable periods, the less frequent the relapse, the less severe it is when it happens, and the shorter its duration. Active monitoring is critical to identifying early signs of relapse; rapid response interventions can prevent worsening.

In severe and persistent mental illnesses the out-of-control phase is characterized by psychosis with delusions, hallucinations, and bizarre behavior. Fortunately, there are an increasing number of available medications that can effectively reduce the out-of-control phase in a matter of days to a few weeks, at most, for the vast majority of people.

When someone is admitted to a traditional psychiatric hospital, the institution provides for all basic needs: a place to live, food, health care, recreational and social activities, etc. Moreover, the staff operate three shifts a day, seven days a week, to ensure that all these needs are provided for the patient. Once the individual is discharged, however, a dramatic change in the intensity of care usually occurs. Although needs continue to be broad and varied, only limited services are provided by clinicians outside the hospital. The person faces the task of living in the community alone, without staff support. Even when a detailed discharge plan including all the requirements has been made, the person no longer has a team of professionals to ensure that those requirements will be met. The consequence of this marked reduction of services when in the community is that a person discharged from a mental hospital has a 60 percent chance of being readmitted within two years. Some further statistics highlight this fact: In the United States over the last twenty-five years, the number of patients placed from state hospitals into the community has risen dramatically, accompanied by a dramatic increase in readmission rates to mental hospitals, from about 150,000 patients to about 400,000 yearly. In essence, what was accomplished was the replacement of one inadequate mode of care (keeping people institutionalized for long periods) with another inadequate mode of care (having patients revolve in and out of the hospital). Under the current system, the patient comes into the hospital, receives short-term help, is released into the community, runs into new problems, has a new crisis, and has to be readmitted.

A logical question to ask about this pattern is this: Why can't the typical severely mentally ill person function successfully in the community after release from the hospital? On discharge, the individual has been stabilized and relieved of many of the severe symptoms of the illness. Thus, he or she is no longer psychotic and has a good discharge plan that includes the prerequisites to "make it" in the community. Why, then, can he or she not organize and maintain for himself or herself the necessities of life, the way people without a mental illness do? The answer involves issues to which we have not paid sufficient attention.

In spite of optimal medication regimens, many people with these illnesses continue to suffer from significant long-term impairments, which result from a combination of factors, including negative symptoms of the illness, persistent positive symptoms, character pathology, and organic pathology. Whatever their cause, these impairments seriously interfere with the capacity to maintain a stable adjustment in the community without support. These long-term impairments include the following:

1. A high vulnerability to stress (a small amount of stress can cause extreme anxiety and psychosis);
2. Difficulty with interpersonal relationships;
3. Deficiency in basic coping skills (e.g., the ability to shop in a supermarket, use public transportation, budget money);
4. Marked dependency (it is not unusual to have been dependent on hospitals or family for long periods of time);
5. Poor transfer of learning.

The problem with transfer of learning is particularly significant. It has been found that even when a substantial amount of time is spent in the hospital teaching people the skills they will need to live in the community, they do not use these skills after discharge. This is, in part, because they have difficulty generalizing what they have learned in the hospital to the new community setting. Perhaps even more significantly, many people with severe and persistent mental illness find that anything new is highly stressful. Therefore, they tend to avoid new situations and new experiences, even though they may have mastered the skills required to cope with the new situation.

It cannot be emphasized too strongly that these long-term impairments interfere with a person's ability to organize and maintain the necessities required to develop a sustained and adequate life in the community. We found that, even when good discharge plans are made, the person's long-term impairments are major impediments to following through on those plans. The following examples illustrate this.

Example 1. Keeping the post-discharge appointment at the community mental health center in order to renew the medication prescription. On the day and the time of his appointment, the clinician at the center went into the waiting room and called the person's name. He was not there. The clinician went back to his office and said to himself, "It is too bad that the he is not motivated enough to follow through on his treatment plan, but I certainly can use the time to catch up on my paperwork."

In fact, the individual in question wanted very much to follow through on his discharge plan and he faithfully took his medication every day. However, on the day of his mental health center appointment he was too anxious to go. Upon questioning him, we learned that his anxiety was secondary to two factors: One, he did not know which bus to take to the center and even if he got on the right bus, he did not know when to get off; secondly, and more importantly, he was very anxious about meeting a new clinician he had never seen before and having to tell that new person his whole history.

Thus it was not his lack of motivation that got in the way of following through with his discharge plans; rather, it was the long-term impairments of his illness that prevented him from keeping his center appointment. Specifically, he didn't have the coping skills to figure out his bus route, the deficit in his interpersonal skills made it difficult for him to meet and confide in a new clinician, and, very importantly, significant anxiety was created by having to do several new tasks (going to a new center, seeing new people, and figuring out his bus route). All these factors, acting together, blocked his ability to follow through on his discharge plans. All of this could have been easily overcome if he had had someone who would take him to his first few appointments and even, if necessary, sit in the appointments with him. The consequence of not having this service available led to the inevitable: He ran out of medication and, in a relatively short time, was once again psychotic and readmitted to the hospital.

Example 2. Having sufficient money to live in the community. Prior to discharge, care was taken that the patient's SSI check would be sent to his new place of residence; thus, he indeed received his check at the beginning of each month. The patient knew a great deal about music and the electronic equipment necessary to obtain high fidelity. On the fifteenth of the month, he happened to pass an electronics store and saw the exact equipment he had been hoping to have someday; he went in and purchased it. As a result, he spent all his money and would not be receiving any more until the next month, some two weeks hence. Within two days, his refrigerator was empty and he was out of food; he was beside himself with worry, and within a short time he was again experiencing psychotic symptoms and was readmitted to the hospital.

The major reason he ran out of money was not that he was frivolous; it was because of the deficiency in his coping skills to budget his monthly income, a consequence of a long-term impairment of his mental illness. All this could have been avoided if he had had someone who was monitoring him closely enough to know when he was out of money. That person could have taken him to the welfare office to get enough money to get him through the month until his check came. In addition, he could then have gotten help learning how to budget his money and, if necessary, help in managing the money on a daily basis.

Example 3. Having a place to live. During his hospitalization, the patient lost his place of residence, a not-infrequent occurrence. The discharge plan included a new place to live and an appointment at a psychosocial rehabilitation clubhouse where he could spend time during the day and be involved in a rehabilitation program. Following discharge from the hospital, he did not go to the clubhouse because of the long-term impairments similar to those described in the first example. He began to sleep later and later during the day and stay up until the early hours in the morning. He spent most of his time watching TV or listening to music. Unfortunately, he did these activities with the volume turned up quite high. The neighbors began to complain and he was warned several times by the landlord that this had to change or he would be evicted. Because of the long-term impairment of poor interpersonal skills, he did not negotiate with the landlord or make peace with his neighbors and, as a result, he was evicted. After a few days of wandering the streets with no place to live, he was again experiencing psychotic symptoms and, within a short time, was readmitted to the hospital.

Again, all of this could have been avoided if he had had someone closely monitoring his functioning and intervening when needed: He could have had help working things out with his landlord and neighbors; he could have had someone accompany him to the clubhouse until he was comfortable being there; he could have had a headset purchased for him, so that when he did listen to TV or music in the late hours he would not be disturbing others.

Example 4. Utilizing skills learned while in the hospital. While in the hospital, patients were taught how to shop in a supermarket by taking them to the supermarket near the hospital. They were also taught how to prepare simple meals in the model kitchen the hospital had for that purpose. On discharge, however, we found that many of the clients were not shopping or cooking but instead were buying their meals in fast-food restaurants. When they were asked why, a not-unusual response was, "I went to the supermarket in my neighborhood and I couldn't find what I was looking for. I walked up and down the aisles looking and then noticed that people were staring at me and whispering about me. And so I left, and didn't return." We all have had the experience of going into a strange supermarket. It is difficult to find things and it is somewhat anxiety-provoking; however, we generally bind our anxiety and find most of what we need. For these clients, however, the long-term impairments reduced their capacity to cope, which increased their anxiety level, and they soon found themselves experiencing a return of psychotic thinking. People were not, in fact, staring or whispering about them.

These examples illustrate how the long-term impairments of the illness interfere with the clients' ability to organize and maintain the prerequisites to a stable adjustment to life in the community. The chapters that follow describe intervention strategies and guiding principles to help clients with serious and persistent mental illness live in the community with the rest of us, where there is the potential and opportunity to give meaning to life.

Suggested Readings

Jamison, K. R. (1995). *An unquiet mind: A memoir of mood and madness.* New York: Knopf.

Mechanic, D., & Aiken, L. H. (1987). Improving the care of patients with chronic mental illness. *New England Journal of Medicine, 317,* 1634–1638.

Stein, L. I., & Diamond, R. J. (1985). A program for difficult to treat patients. *New Directions for Mental Health Services, 26* , 17–26.

Stroul, B. A. (1989). Community support systems for persons with long-term mental illness: A conceptual network. *Psychosocial Rehabilitation Journal, 12,* 9–26.

Test, M. A. (1992). Training in community living. In R. P. Liberman (Ed.), *Handbook of Psychiatric Rehabilitation.* New York: Macmillan.

Turner, J. C., & TenHoor, W. J. (1978). The NIMH community support program: Pilot approach to a needed social reform. *Schizophrenia Bulletin, 4,* 319–328.

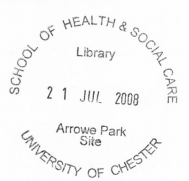

6

The Continuous Care Strategy

Community mental health treatment is sometimes referred to as "aftercare." This term erroneously connotes that the important treatment phase takes place in the hospital, and then, following discharge, the less important care takes place in the community. To say the least, community care is often woefully inadequate. People routinely receive intensive services while hospitalized but very little care following discharge to help them remain stable. Unfortunately, our current funding mechanisms support this pattern of care.

This inappropriate approach is probably unique to the care of persons with mental illnesses and would not be tolerated if these individuals were not so stigmatized by society. No one would consider using such an episode-oriented approach (treating the disease only when it gets out of control) as the treatment strategy for other chronic illnesses such as diabetes or chronic heart disease. Everyone recognizes that those diseases, and similar physical diseases, require a continuous-care strategy outside the hospital in order for patients to remain stable and to maintain their functional capacity.

To successfully stabilize chronic mental and physical conditions continuous monitoring and treatment are required. Continuous care strategies are employed with chronic diseases that are incurable but manageable. This strategy is the keystone to helping persons with severe and persistent mental illness make a satisfactory life in the community and provides services on a continuing basis. It is not good enough to claim you are providing "continuity of care" and "coordination of services" by simply having communications among different service providers. For too many people this approach simply will not work. The continuous care strategy is directed toward the task of helping the person make a stable life of decent quality in the community. It accomplishes this through the following four functions.

1. *The utilization of a broad approach.* This means that the ACT team focuses

on any and all factors that impact on the person's stability in the community, including those that will interfere with or facilitate that stability. These factors include the following: finances, living arrangements, activities of daily living, socialization, vocational and/or avocational activities, crisis resolution services, medical services, and mental health services. Most of the services are delivered by the ACT team. When appropriate, the team brokers for some services; for example, it typically finds and develops a relationship with a physician to provide general medical services and does the same with landlords to provide housing.

2. *Acting as the fixed point of responsibility for all aspects of the person's life that affect his or her stability in the community.* Translated, this means that, even if someone else is providing a service, the ACT team assumes the responsibility to ensure it is being done well. To accomplish this, it carefully monitors the provision of that service: If it is not going well, it tries to help the provider do a better job; if that is not possible, it finds a new provider; and if that can't be done, it provides the service itself. The bottom line is that, if a client needs a service, the ACT team is the responsible entity for making sure it is provided.

3. *Careful monitoring.* The team must know what is going on in a person's life so that it can intervene promptly to help. The importance of careful monitoring cannot be overemphasized. One critical function of careful monitoring is to be aware of impending relapse as early as possible, so that rapid intervention may be employed to prevent a full-blown psychotic episode. One very useful technique in this regard is to be aware of what the early signs of relapse are for each person. This varies greatly from person to person and can present in a variety of ways. For example, it may begin with difficulty sleeping or becoming suspicious of others. For most, the early signs remain quite constant; in other words, there is a good bit of variability between people but quite a bit of constancy in any given person—that is, prior to each relapse, the individual would experience the same early signs unique to him. Therefore, it is important for the team, in its initial assessment as well as ongoing assessments, to learn the early signs of relapse for each individual. The next step is to help the client become aware of these signs and to report them to the team as soon as perceived. Also, with the client's permission, it is very useful to teach the early signs to those who are close to the client and in frequent contact with him.

Once the client becomes aware of his early signs and reports them promptly, treating that client to prevent relapse becomes enormously easier. However, one must not become discouraged if it does not happen quickly. It is difficult for most people not to rationalize away the early signs of any illness. It is especially difficult not to rationalize signs of mental illness, since it is such a stigmatizing disorder. Thus, it may be necessary to experience several relapses before learning the importance of self-monitoring for early signs. Of course, monitoring for all the client's needs is a crucial team function; in the next chapter, on the nuts and bolts of operating a team, a detailed description of how this monitoring is done will be provided.

4. *There are no arbitrary time limits on how long a person will be served by the team or on how long any specific service will be provided.* The concept is that the team or the specific intervention will be provided as long as the user can benefit or until another alternative would be better. This concept was introduced by the original ACT research. Prior to that time, it was standard procedure that all services, other than medication, were to be time-limited. As an example, when a patient was discharged from a hospital and was sent to a halfway house, the halfway house usually had a three-month or six-month time limit, after which the person had to leave, whether ready or not. This approach assumed that all people would be able to move "upward" after a certain length of time in that "treatment" setting. All interventions were conceptualized as treatments, not as supports, and virtually no consideration was given to individual differences.

In addition, the prevalent strategy was one of moving people through a series of settings, from more to less structure. Little consideration was given to providing more normalized living situations as well as immediate onsite support to ensure that the person could be successful in that setting. No consideration was given to the stress involved in moving from one setting to another, which, in many cases, is greater than the stress of being in a less structured setting initially. This same time-limited thinking was utilized in delivery of virtually all other services, from day treatment to vocational rehabilitation. The ACT research clearly showed that services may have to be provided over long periods of time and, in some cases, a lifetime; further, it suggested that many of these interventions are better conceptualized as needed supports rather than treatments. This does not imply that clients should not be moved to either more or less structured settings; rather, the concept is that no a priori time limits are set, that all decisions are based on individual assessments and, when possible, transitions should be made gradually.

Continuous Care via Single Person or Team?

In an attempt to rectify the problem of fragmentation in community services, the "case manager" model was developed. This model utilized a single person to carry a caseload and to act as the "glue" in the system by working with all area service providers to ensure that everyone received the services needed and did not fall through the cracks and get lost in the system. This model borrowed heavily from the early ACT research but tried to accomplish the same tasks by using a single person instead of a team and by giving that person a much higher caseload than utilized by the ACT approach. Only in a system that has a rich supply of services might this work and then only for some of those intended. The single case manager model does not work well for those who are resistant to being treated or who require more intense support and help than one clinician can provide.

People may object to being referred to as "cases" and as being "managed"; these terms treat persons as objects and infer passivity on their part in the whole treatment process. We recommend using terms that do not suffer from that problem, such as "care coordinator" or "primary contact person." In ACT work, we prefer "primary contact person" because it implies that other members of the ACT team are also involved with each team member's individual caseload. It is the term that is most consistent with the team approach, which is so crucial to the operation of the ACT program. However, the reader should recognize that in the ACT literature the term "case manager" is ubiquitous.

It must be stressed that in the ACT model the whole team remains responsible for the care of the each client and every member of the team is involved, at one time or another, with virtually every client. However, to take lead responsibility for each person and be responsible for follow-through and advocacy, each ACT team member (except the secretary and part-time psychiatrist) serves as a primary contact person for a portion of that team's roster. The number of people carried by the various primary contact persons varies according to other responsibilities that they may have. When using this model, care must be taken to ensure that there is a good match between the primary contact person and the respective service recipient. Both personal and professional variables should be taken into consideration. For example, if a man feels competitive with other men and does not get along with them, a woman may be chosen. If someone has significant medical problems and a good understanding of the physical illness and medical treatments is required, a nurse may be chosen. When using this model, the first primary contact person assignment should be considered tentative. After the staff person gets to know the person well, it may be decided that someone else would be more effective; then, with the participation of the targeted person, the transition is made from one to the other (the staff person should not be chosen simply because he or she is "next up"). Of course, equitable distribution of clients among the staff must be maintained, but it should be done in a way to maximize, as much as possible, the naturally occurring "best fit" between staff person and client.

Some ACT programs don't designate primary contact persons, not even for administrative tasks. This is done to emphasize that, in ACT, case management functions are shared by the full team. Whether the team utilizes a primary contact person or not, every member of the team is involved on a regular basis with every person. This model serves their long-term treatment and rehabilitation needs, which require staff to maintain productive relationships over long periods of time. While a single clinician cannot promise availability for a lifelong supportive relationship, a team can, with some certainty, assure that the team is committed to working with the service recipient on a long-term basis. Such a commitment provides an anchor in the community for people in a pattern of repeated hospitalizations and failed living arrangements. The long-term trusting relationship with the team becomes a vehicle for change, in and of itself.

Table 6-1 lists the duties of the primary contact person; for the most part, these duties have an administrative and coordinating function. However, it cannot be stressed too strongly that in the ACT model, all team members are ultimately responsible for the carrying out of these duties, for, in fact, all team members will be involved with virtually all the clients.

Table 6-1
Duties of the Primary Contact Person on the ACT Team

- Serves as the primary monitor of his or her clients' functioning and communicates that to other staff.
- Ensures that clients receive benefits for which they are eligible.
- Ensures that client records are kept current; prepares the narrative developed in treatment planning meetings; schedules treatment planning and other special meetings involving the client; makes sure that any paperwork required for the client is completed on time; etc.
- Leads and facilitates the treatment planning process, including the initial treatment plan, the first comprehensive treatment plan, and the six-month update plans.
- Leads the discussion at staff meetings regarding the client to ensure that the client's various needs are addressed at those meetings.
- Locates and monitors all necessary medical, social, and psychiatric services that cannot be provided by the ACT team.
- Ensures that clients have adequate housing in the most normalized setting possible.
- Assists in the development and execution of a plan for assuring income maintenance.
- Assists in connecting clients to appropriate social networks.
- Provides much of the direct contact for his or her clients, such as accompanying them to appointments and helping them with daily living activities (apartment upkeep, shopping, laundry, etc.).
- Assists with any other activities that are necessary to maintain psychiatric stability in a community-based setting.

Crisis Stabilization and the Proper Use of Hospital Services

The ACT team expends most of its effort helping people maintain stability in the community, especially when the program is young and many of the clients are new to the program. When an individual is in crisis, the team helps him or her resolve the crisis in the shortest time possible and in the least restrictive environment. The ACT team serves as the gatekeeper for hospitalization. When someone's condition is so out of control that hospitalization is necessary, an ACT team member accompanies the individual to the hospital and helps him or her and the hospital staff know what is hoped will be accomplished by the hospital stay. When a client must be hospitalized, the ACT team works closely with the inpatient staff on treatment and discharge planning, keeps the person's support system intact, gets him or her back into the community as quickly as possible, and then shifts back to a continuous treatment strategy to provide comprehensive care in the community.

As noted in the previous section, close monitoring is crucial so that successful early intervention can prevent a full-blown relapse. As soon as the team becomes aware that the person is in crisis, the response must be as quick as possible. That is why twenty-four-hour availability is so important. The first step is to carefully assess the individual in his or her context and learn the circumstances that precipitated the crisis. The assessment of the individual will help in making a decision as to how much supervision will be required to get through the crisis. Learning the circumstances that precipitated the crisis will help in determining what environmental manipulations need to be made in order to stabilize the situation.

As noted above, when working with a person in crisis it is important to see the crisis in its context. This is best done by going to where the crisis is happening, which not infrequently is the person's place of living. This approach will not only help the clinician more effectively resolve the crisis but also enhance the probability that the person will be able to remain where he is and thus experience as little disruption in his life as possible. For example, with an episode of interpersonal conflict between the client and others he is living with, frequently the client will be the one who appears most distraught and displays pathological behavior. However, by conceptualizing the problem as a group situation and intervening with the entire group, it is often possible to resolve the situation so that he or she will be able to remain at home. There are occasions, however, when the interpersonal situation is so hot that the person must leave the field in order to restabilize. Once outside of the turbulent situation, he or she may stabilize quite quickly. Then the task is to find a place for him or her to stay for a few days until things cool down back home. Developing a relationship with a hotel or motel manager for just such purposes is very useful. The manager is assured that the bill will be paid and that an ACT staff person will be available twenty-four hours a day to respond, on site, if there are any problems. Likewise, the client is given the telephone number of the ACT person to call anytime, day or night, if he is having a problem. Of course, the ACT person will be seen early the next morning and as frequently as needed during this crisis period. Having a resource like that available has several advantages. It provides a normalized solution to the problem, the individual can remain on his job or involved with other community activities, and it is very cost-effective. If the person is too disturbed to utilize the hotel and requires a more supervised setting, then the use of community emergency beds or the hospital is necessary.

The relationship of the ACT staff with the staff of the crisis bed unit and the hospital unit is of crucial importance. The relationship must be one of collaboration, with the ACT team playing an active role while clients are in those facilities. In the first place, the ACT staff serves as the gatekeeper to all admissions. Thus, when the ACT team determines that a client cannot be managed in the community and requires admission, a good relationship with the inpatient staff will greatly facilitate that process. An ACT staff member should accompany the person to the unit, ensure that all pertinent information is given to the inpatient staff, including, specifically, what the ACT team expects to have happen as a result of the admission. This may include a reduction in specific target signs and symptoms, having family sessions, etc. During the stay, the ACT team should visit the inpatient daily, be involved in treatment planning with the ward staff, and, when appropriate (even while on inpatient status), keep the patient involved with community activities to the greatest degree possible.

While the patient is hospitalized, the ACT team should do everything possible to keep the client's community supports intact so that they will be available upon discharge. For example, with the client's permission, his or her family and significant other would be kept abreast of his or her condition; the person's employer would be alerted that the employee is sick and told approximately when he or she will be returning to work; and, if the person's rent becomes due, it would be paid so that the living situation would be kept intact, etc. These activities keep a person's community system "glued" together while he or she is in the hospital and, in fact, replace all the discharge planning ordinarily done by the inpatient staff. In essence, the hospital's discharge plan and time of discharge are provided to inpatient staff by the ACT team. This makes good clinical sense, since the ACT team is the clinical entity that will be the major provider of services post-discharge and is involved with the patient and the community during the hospitalization.

A good working relationship with the inpatient staff will greatly increase the probability that they will look to the ACT team to advise them about discharge plans. Gaining inpatient staff cooperation will most certainly happen if the ACT staff relate to the inpatient staff in a respectful manner and stay involved with the case, as described above, during the hospitalization. The most difficult jobs the inpatient team encounters with their patients are getting good information at the time of admission and making truly achievable dispositional plans; the latter is particularly difficult. The ACT team can provide both of these for the inpatient staff, which in itself will go a long way toward developing a good working relationship with the inpatient team.

The hospital is the most expensive cost center in mental health budgets. The cost-effectiveness of the ACT model is directly linked to its ability to reduce hospital use; therefore, using the hospital as efficiently as possible is a major objective of the ACT program. These outcomes are consistent with the goals of modern health-care administrators because the cost of inpatient treatments has become prohibitive. In addition to being cost-effective, efficient use of the hospital makes good clinical sense; clearly, the longer people stay in inpatient facilities, the more difficult it is to reintegrate them into their homes and communities.

Conclusions

Both the hospital and the community are essential in the overall treatment of persons with severe and persistent mental illness. We know, now, that the old debate as to whether the hospital or the community is most important is not a useful exercise. The important questions are, what can best be accomplished in the hospital and what can best be accomplished in the community? It is clear that, while the client is in the community, continuous care is the strategy that will facilitate a stable and satisfactory life and, at the same time, reduce the frequency, duration, and severity of relapse.

In summary, chronic diseases, including chronic mental disorders, require a continuous treatment strategy that is designed to help individuals remain stable, increase functional capacity, and achieve a decent quality of life. To accomplish this, the ACT team serves as the fixed point of responsibility for all needs. There are no arbitrary time limits; that is, services are provided for as long as needed. Services encompass a broad range of needs, including close monitoring, so that the appropriate intervention can be provided quickly.

Suggested Readings

Stein, L. I. (1992). Innovating against the current: Innovative community mental health programs. *New Directions for Mental Health Services, 56.*

Stein, L. I., & Diamond, R. J. (1985). A program for difficult-to-treat patients. *New Directions for Mental Health Services, 26,* 17–26.

Stein, L. I., & Test, M. A. (1976). Retraining hospital staff for work in a community program in Wisconsin. *Hospital and Community Psychiatry, 27,* 266–268.

Torrey, F. E. (1986). Continuous treatment teams in the care of the chronic mentally ill. *Hospital and Community Psychiatry , 37,* 1243–1247.

··●⟩⟩ 7 ⟨⟨⟨··

The ACT Team

The ACT team is the heart of the ACT program. One cannot overemphasize the importance of operating as a real team rather than as a group of individuals calling themselves a team. This chapter describes and discusses: (1) the nature of team interactions and desirable characteristics of all team members; (2) the individual members of the ACT team; (3) team size, caseloads, and model adherence; and (4) teamwork, influence and leadership.

The Nature of Team Interactions and Desirable Characteristics of All Team Members

Ideally, all team members should possess characteristics that facilitate the performance of a range of necessary functions. The nature of in vivo treatment (providing direct services in a natural setting rather than in an office or hospital) requires that staff possess the skills necessary to facilitate community integration. To this end, personal characteristics such as patience, empathy, optimism, persuasiveness, pragmatism, flexibility, good judgment, and "street smarts" are highly desirable.

ACT staff practice a "multi-service" case management approach. An environment that promotes a generic staff identity as "generalists" is desirable. As a generalist, a nurse must be willing to sit in a food stamp office, a counselor must be able to detect medication side effects producing functional limitations, and a physician must be willing to become familiar with the patient beyond the confines of the traditional "medication check." Therefore, members of the staff should possess personal characteristics that enable them to work well in a team setting where responsibilities are shared.

Although professional expertise is important, the professionals on the team must not feel that their expertise can only belong to, and be administered by, themselves. The usual division of labor common to hospital multidisciplinary program staff is, in fact, contraindicated. Rather, a premium is placed on stable, predictable, around-the-clock availability of staff for patients (staff assume responsibility for after-hour direct care and advocacy with landlords, hospitals, local law enforcement personnel, etc.; therefore, potential staff must not be adverse to shift work or to occasional overtime or "off time" work). More often than not, a telephone or in-person intervention by someone whom the patient knows well can interrupt a behavioral pattern that might proceed to crisis proportions. Often, such interventions simply involve questions about medications or reassurance in matters of independent living. When such efforts are lacking, patients who are well-known to treatment programs can turn up as strangers in emergency rooms and be routed off to institutional programs.

Clearly, the continuous care approach encourages formation of a stronger therapeutic alliance than is possible through crisis intervention or brief episodic care. A long-term perspective facilitates early identification of symptom recurrence by staff, clients, and family, which guides medication adjustment or other interventions in a timely fashion. Hence, clinicians should possess the capacity for close observation, as well as curiosity and vigilance about specific symptoms of the illness over the long term. Staff will be teaching other team members, learning from them, and providing education, direction, and encouragement to mentally ill persons and their families.

Active involvement in a person's life, as happens with ACT, is sometimes criticized as "fostering dependence" by office-based therapists who might, for example, assume that tracking down a patient who didn't keep an appointment will only encourage the patient to rely on staff members unnecessarily. They argue that visiting patients in their homes or providing transportation for important appointments will only create dependence and slow the treatment process. These constructs are not helpful in the treatment of individuals with disorders such as schizophrenia and other psychotic disorders. Assertive outreach is critical to the care of these clients because their capacity to function in an organized fashion has been disabled. On the other hand, such relationships require that staff possess both the capacity for intimacy and the capacity to maintain clear professional boundaries. Therefore, all staff must be carefully screened, monitored, and supervised around these important interpersonal issues.

The Individual Members of the ACT Team

Support Staff, the Secretary/Receptionist

The ACT team's secretary is much more than a clerical person. The secretary, as the only team member who is in the office at all times, acts as the interface between the team and the rest of the community, as well as interacting extensively with the clients. In this position, the secretary is a key person in setting the tone for the ACT team's work site. It is important that the clients, as well as the community at large, perceive the ACT team as approachable and welcoming. The more clients feel welcomed, the more likely it is that they will want to be active participants in the process. Thus, in addition to having clerical skills, the secretary must be a mature person, have a friendly disposition, have good interpersonal skills, and exercise good judgment.

The routine duties of the secretary include acting as receptionist—greeting people as they come into ACT, answering the phone and taking messages, typing, and filing. The secretary also has the responsibility of ensuring that the charts are kept up-to-date, making up new charts, and keeping the face sheet updated (address change, phone number change, etc.). The secretary also keeps track of when entries need to be made and, if they are late, sends reminders to staff to produce them. For example, treatment plan updates must be done every six months. The secretary prepares a calendar showing whose treatment plans need updating within the next two months, so that staff can sign up for a treatment planning meeting within the appropriate time span. The secretary then tracks the process and, if necessary, reminds the staff person to complete the updated treatment plan so that it can be filed in the chart.

In many programs, the secretary also manages the finances. This might include routine ACT team expenses such as utility bills, phone bills, and managing the cash fund that is set aside for emergency use. Money management is a critically important part of the ACT program. In many programs, it is the secretary who has the responsibility of putting the money in envelopes for disbursement, paying bills for certain clients, arranging and paying for food vouchers for those requiring them. This money management must be done in a scrupulous and exceedingly careful manner. The secretary may also give prepackaged medications to patients who come in to get them.

The secretary has a great deal of interaction with clients and is in a position not only to be useful to them but also to make observations about clients useful to the staff. Not infrequently, the client receives a letter from an agency that he or she finds confusing. He or she may become worried and want immediate clarification; since the secretary is always in the ACT office, he or she gets the call. Over time, the secretary and the client get to know each other very well.

Other interactions are not routine; for instance, clients may come in or call when distressed and, if a staff person is not available, appeal to the secretary to handle the situation. The more information the secretary has about the client, the more prepared he or she will be to manage the situation for the benefit of the client. The secretary must be able to make judgments about what he or she can manage and to know when the situation is beyond his or her ability, that is, when to immediately contact the primary staff person.

The importance of the secretary being thoroughly knowledgeable about clients cannot be overemphasized. It is critical that the secretary regularly attend staff meetings where clients are discussed, for, in addition to getting information, the secretary will be able to contribute a good deal learned from his or her interactions with clients.

Social Workers

Social workers are trained as generalists and so make ideal ACT team members. The well trained social worker has clinical skills and a broad perspective in their utilization. The social worker also has knowledge about the resources that are needed by the clients and ensures that they get them. This requires familiarity with the various bureaucracies and how to get things accomplished within them. Each bureaucracy has its own idiosyncratic maze, within which the social worker needs to know how to maneuver. These include financial agencies such as Supplemental Security Income (SSI), Social Security Disability Income (SSDI), General Assistance, etc., and the judicial system, with district attorneys, public defenders, parole and probation officers, and the writing of reports required by them and the court. The social worker must know how to write necessary reports and procure guardians when needed. He or she must have the knowledge to work with housing authorities and be familiar with federal, state, and local regulations. In addition, the well trained social worker has the clinical skills to provide counseling services to clients, provide psychoeducational services to families, and work with the children of clients, where knowledge about a whole cadre of different agencies is necessary. Social workers on ACT teams generally serve as the primary contact person for a full load of clients (about twelve).

Nursing

Virtually every client served by an ACT team takes psychiatric medications, which have side effects and interact with other medications the client may be taking. Since the psychiatrist is part-time, nurses must have the expertise to play a central role in pharmacologic management. All staff are cross-trained to be familiar with psychiatric medications and their side effects; when such effects are noticed, they are brought to the attention of the nurse. If the situation requires rapid action, the psychiatrist can be called and a telephone order can be given to the nurse to change the medication dosage or type. The nurse also gives depot medication injections, reviews the lab results, and packages medications. In addition, the nurse monitors physical medical problems as directed by the physician. For example, the nurse may monitor blood pressure, weight, the presence or absence of edema, etc. As the liaison between the primary care physician and the patient, the nurse will take the patient to appointments, sit in on the consultation, and then help the patient understand what the doctor said, thus helping with follow through on the doctor's orders. The nurse is often the primary contact person for those ACT recipients who have significant medical problems. The number of clients for which the nurse serves as primary contact person varies from team to team, depending on how much of the above medical work needs to done. Typically, the nurse does not carry a full load and has about eight clients for whom he or she is the primary contact person.

The Psychologist

The psychologist, as a broadly trained mental health professional, can be a valuable member of the team. Typically, like the social worker, the psychologist serves as a generalist on the team and carries a full caseload (primary contact person for about twelve clients). The psychologist, trained in a broad array of psychotherapies, uses his or her skills in individual, group, and family work, as well as in crisis resolution. The psychologist is especially useful in helping to develop behavior therapy programs to address specific client problems.

The Vocational Specialist

The vocational specialist must be trained in supported employment, the vocational rehabilitation approach used in the context of ACT. Along with other staff, the vocational specialist assists the client in developing job skills at the actual employment site while monitoring his acclimation to the job with regard to attendance, performance of job functions, and social skills required in the employment setting. This involves a combination of teaching, advocacy, and mediation. The employment specialist provides as much and whatever type of support and assistance the client needs to obtain and keep a job or to move on to another job. Vocational assessment is a continuous process; that is, each work experience adds knowledge about the client's interest and abilities. The vocational specialist helps the client integrate these experiences and use them to make the next step more successful. The role of the vocational specialist on the ACT team is discussed in more detail in Chapter 10.

Drug and Alcohol Use Specialist

Having a specialist in alcohol and drug use as a member of the ACT team greatly enhances the team's effectiveness. Over half of persons with severe mental illness in the U.S. develop problems with the use of alcohol and/or illicit drugs during their lives. The use of psychoactive substances destabilizes mental illness and interferes with rehabilitation.

Thus, clients in ACT services receive substance abuse and mental health treatment in an integrated fashion, rather than in the traditional approach that treats these conditions separately. When substance abuse services are provided in the context of ACT, problems with compliance and "treatment dropout" are reduced. The ACT team's focus on assisting clients with basic needs augments the significance of the therapeutic relationship and provides for greater motivation/leverage for behavioral change.

The drug and alcohol use specialists on ACT teams must be familiar with problems related to the use of street drugs in this population, and must possess the clinical skills necessary to engage patients in treatment. In addition, they must be proficient at delivering specific substance abuse interventions: acute detoxification strategies, the use of pharmacological adjuncts, strategies that involve well-structured "talking therapies," social and environmental strategies, and strategies that employ more coercion and/or external controls. Chapter 10 discusses in greater detail how substance abuse specialists work with these clients in the context of ACT teamwork.

The Psychiatrist

Psychiatrists are more likely than other staff to work part-time or to be assigned part-time to several teams. The psychiatrist is often the only member of the team who is not employed full-time to work with a given team's caseload. Thus, the psychiatrist is not always present when team members come together to share information or make decisions. Since the psychiatrist is frequently not present and so does not hear all of the information firsthand, the other team staff members are constantly making decisions about what information to pass on to the psychiatrist and what issues the psychiatrist should be involved with.

How well the psychiatrist can function as an integrated part of the team depends on the skills of the psychiatrist, as well as the attitudes of the other team members toward him or her. This is often complicated by the psychiatrist's difficulty in finding a comfortable place in the team hierarchy. Most psychiatrists are uncomfortable with the idea of having a nonphysician as their "boss." This is as much a cultural and political problem as a clinical one, but many psychiatrists feel that only another M.D. can truly understand and supervise their medical decisions. What happens if a psychiatrist who is medically responsible for a clinical decision disagrees with his or her team leader? In a well functioning team, with a skilled team leader and a skilled psychiatrist, unresolvable disagreement does not occur. When important disagreements do occur, additional information is collected, the pros and cons of each solution are considered, and new options are pursued until a plan can be developed that everyone can support. Teams do not always function ideally, however, and even psychiatrists who are comfortable with a nonmedical team leader generally prefer some way of structuring their role so that they are formally supervised by another physician with whom they can share legal responsibility.

One alternative is for the psychiatrist to be neither above nor below the team leader but to have his or her own supervisory structure outside of the one for nonmedical staff. The Mental Health Center of Dane County operates with this kind of parallel hierarchy. Each clinical program has a team leader who is responsible for running the team and supervising the clinical staff and a team medical director who is administratively co-equal to the team leader but who has no formal administrative authority. This system functions extremely well in Dane County, in large part because the medical directors of each team and the team leaders have been able to negotiate their inherently ambiguous relationship with each other.

An ACT team should have at least twenty hours a week of one psychiatrist's time. Being a part-time team member makes it difficult to be perceived as integral and this, in turn, limits how much the psychiatrist can contribute. Expertise about medical illnesses and medications is essential, but if this is all that is addressed by the team psychiatrist it will indeed reinforce the perception of a narrow role. The more the psychiatrist can put medication issues into the larger context of the client's life, the more useful he or she will be to clients and other staff. In addition, psychiatrists can increase the team's effectiveness by teaching the nonmedical team members about medications and their side effects. Psychiatrists often have access to upper-level managers and can help make management aware of policies that interfere with clinical work. This kind of intervention can improve the overall work environment and satisfaction of other mental health professionals. The psychiatrist's status also means that his or her praise or criticism of another clinician may carry special weight in that person's annual review, promotion, or general professional reputation.

For effective and efficient ACT work, the psychiatrist must be available and accessible. A psychiatrist who is readily available is more likely to increase a fellow team member's sense of effectiveness. This, in turn, increases the likelihood that the psychiatrist will be sought out in the future. Availability requires both physical and psychological accessibility—being physically present or easily reachable and being helpful and collegial rather than dictatorial and demeaning. The relative shortage of psychiatrists can encourage both the psychiatrist and the team to feel that they are indispensable and irreplaceable. When this factor is perceived positively, the value of the psychiatrist is enhanced. It is important that the psychiatrist be clearly identified as a member of a team; if not, he or she is likely to be left out of the informal information networking that teams use to develop policies and practices that influence how they will work with clients.

There is a direct relationship between the amount of effort the psychiatrist is willing to exert in helping the team function and the amount of influence the psychiatrist will be given as a result of that effort. For example, a psychiatrist who clearly indicates that staff can call him or her after hours will have more influence than one who is perceived as less available. The help a psychiatrist offers may take many forms. Involvement in decisions outside of those perceived as strictly medical indicates more widespread interest in the team. Occasionally coming in over an evening or weekend to see how those shifts operate, being available for emergencies, having lunch with staff rather than off on one's own, attending social affairs—all will facilitate team functioning.

Psychiatrists sometimes assume that they should have power and authority based on their years of training or their status as physicians or that they have ultimate responsibility for all aspects of a client's treatment. In reality, the psychiatrist's influence over other team members usually has to be earned. Psychiatrists can have a large impact, both on the team as an organization and on the treatment of individual clients, but psychiatrists must learn how to behave so that such an impact is possible. Working on an ACT team can be professionally rewarding but requires that interested psychiatrists, in addition to having excellent clinical skills, practice a wide range of effective social and administrative skills. The most important of these is knowing how to exercise informal power and influence so as to have a positive impact on team functioning in ways that beneficially affect the lives of the clients served.

Hiring Clients as Program Staff

In large measure due to federal policies and funding for the development of a range of activities for clients of mental health services, the role of clients as providers of mental health services is receiving increasing attention. The funding emanates from the Community Support Program of the Center for Mental Health Services (CMHS), which is part of the Federal Substance Abuse and Mental Health Service Administration.

Drs. Lisa Dixon, Anthony Lehman, and colleagues at the Baltimore ACT program (a CMHS McKinney-funded research project designed to measure the effectiveness of ACT for homeless persons with severe mental illness) have published very positive impressions of the role of clients as ACT service providers. They note that as staff members they can make valuable contributions to the work of the team by virtue of having learned to successfully cope with their own situations and illnesses. They are clearly in a better position to appreciate daily living problems of other people with severe mental illness and are in a good position to help others with their concerns regarding medications. They can function as true advocates, reminding the team of the service recipient's point of view. Individuals who do not trust the professional members of the ACT team may be more inclined to trust another person suffering from severe mental illness; thus, they may be better able to engage clients who avoid mental health professionals. Their personal experience can also sensitize other staff with regard to numerous issues, including the discomfort produced by side effects of medication. They can serve as constant reminders of the need for education at all levels about mental illness. In addition, they can provide positive role models for other clients and providers alike and can help reduce stigma by challenging staff biases and prejudices.

Team Size, Caseload, and Model Adherence

The original ACT team had eighteen staff, half of whom did not have professional school training and worked as psychiatric aides on the wards of the hospital prior to becoming ACT staff members. Since then, the trend has been toward smaller teams of persons, all of whom (except the secretary) are mental health professionals. The teams in Rhode Island employ a minimum of ten and a maximum of fifteen full-time equivalent (FTE) staff persons with a caseload of no more than ten persons per FTE staff member. The caseload never goes above one hundred and fifty. The Rhode Island teams, in addition to the team leader and part-time psychiatrist, have at least two FTE registered nurses and one or more experienced employment specialists; all remaining staff have achieved at least an associate's degree in the social sciences or equivalent experience.

In the Dane County, Wisconsin, system, the teams tend to be smaller in size—eight team members plus a part-time psychiatrist. Client-to-staff ratio in Wisconsin is generally in the ten-to-one range. Wisconsin has an administrative code with the power of state statute mandating that, in order for ACT services to qualify for reimbursement, staff must fulfill certain educational requirements. Thus, virtually all staff have bachelor's and/or master's degrees. In Wisconsin, ACT teams are termed CSP teams (Community Support Programs), in recognition of federal guidelines about the use of these systems with adults with severe mental illnesses.

Michigan, which has the greatest number of ACT teams in the United States, began with a team size of ten and a caseload of one hundred, but decided that this was too large and now runs with teams of approximately eight with sixty clients, with a staff composition as follows: psychiatrist—eight to twelve hours a week; at least one full-time nurse; at least one master's level social worker or psychologist. The rest of the team is composed of persons with master's or bachelor's degrees in one of the human service areas. In addition, they try to have a staff person who is also a client. Clearly, there is a good deal of variability. It is important to note, however, that teams should not have a client-to-staff ratio of greater than ten-to-one and that a team should not be larger than fifteen FTE persons. In determining the ten-to-one ratio, the psychiatrist and the secretary should not be counted.

The effectiveness of ACT programs may be correlated to model adherence. The Dartmouth ACT Fidelity Scale yields its highest rating for staff composition when, for each set of fifty clients, there is: (1) a half-time psychiatrist; (2) a full-time nurse; (3) a full-time substance abuse specialist; and (4) a full-time vocational rehabilitation counselor.

Although there is a good bit of variability, the important factors are as follows:

1. The team size should be large enough so that there can be coverage seven days a week, with some coverage in the evening hours during the week, and an on-call schedule to ensure a twenty-four hour per day response when needed. We suggest a team no smaller than eight persons, not counting the secretary or psychiatrist.

2. The team should not be so large as to inhibit the development of a close team spirit and good team communication. We suggest a team no larger than twelve persons, not counting the secretary or psychiatrist.

3. The staff should include the trained professionals needed to do the job. We recommend a psychiatrist, nurse, social worker, psychologist, vocational rehabilitation specialist, and drug and alcohol abuse specialist. The team leader may be from any of these professions, but may not substitute for one of them. The numbers of each would be determined by team size, local factors, etc.

4. The great majority of the staff should be full-time; we recommend that no more than 20 percent of the staff be part-time.

5. This is hard, highly responsible work, and it is important to pay people fairly and to offer professional benefits.

6. Staff turnover should be as low as possible. Two factors that greatly reduce turnover are a well functioning team and careful selection during the hiring process. When screening job applicants, one should look for backgrounds in rehabilitation, community home health care, and field-based case management. Although it temporarily increases the burden on the team, it is better to wait and get the right person rather than filling the position quickly. ACT program job descriptions may seem unusual to potential employees trained as traditional office-based outpatient therapists. Be sure to provide clear job descriptions for prospective employees.

7. The client-to-staff ratio should be no lower than eight-to-one and no higher than ten-to-one.

Teamwork, Influence and Leadership

Staff's satisfaction is associated with their capacity to make significant contributions. Therefore, optimizing staff's contributions will lead to improved staff morale and team effectiveness. The level of contribution to the group effort is most evident during "team rounds," where most decisions regarding treatment planning are made. The level of influence a team member has in the decision-making process is based on a variety of factors. The most obvious source of influence is clinical expertise. Also increasing one's influence are availability and longevity within an organization. Availability requires both physical and psychological accessibility—being physically present or easily reachable and being collegial and helpful.

When a team member helps to increase the effectiveness of other members of the team, he or she will come to have greater influence within the team. As a person works in an organization longer, he or she will tend to be connected to more people within the organization, to be more knowledgeable about how things work, and to know more about how to get things done. From this, it follows that people tend to accumulate influence and informal power as their tenure in an organization increases; however, often it is not absolute tenure but relative seniority, that is, a person's tenure compared to that of others on the staff, that is important. The extraordinary power of the staff person who has "been there forever" is well known, as is the relative impotency of the supervisor who has just arrived. Members of an organization gain influence when they are perceived as useful and helpful, so the amount of time a person spends with the team sharing valuable information will certainly affect his or her power.

Being a part-time team member makes it more difficult to influence the team and to be experienced by the team as an integral member. For example, those teams with a stable work force of nonmedical staff but a rapid turnover of psychiatrists will, thus, have psychiatrists who do not have much power or influence. This is an insidious process, since there is likely to be more psychiatrist turnover in teams where psychiatrists feel they have little power to influence decisions; this turnover will lead to psychiatrists who have little real power because of short tenure.

A number of other factors, apart from expertise and instrumental utility, also affect a person's role within an organization. A person will tend to have increased influence if he or she is perceived by other staff as having a commitment to the organization. In general, part-time people are perceived as less committed than full-time staff and temporary staff have less influence than staff who are permanent.

Just as a number of factors can increase one's usefulness and influence within an organization, there are factors that can decrease one's influence. If one alienates other mental health professionals or is perceived as interfering with their effectiveness, one's role will be sabotaged in subtle but powerful ways. Team members who withhold information from their colleagues, who are not reliably available, or who consistently seek praise and attention for themselves will tend to be excluded from their team. They will miss being given important information about a client, suggestions they make will be ignored or misinterpreted, they will tend to be excluded from important discussions about program planning, and they will see both their influence and their effectiveness diminish.

The Team Leader

Having a competent team leader is crucial to team functioning. The team and the clients work closely over a protracted period of time and, in a real way, are like a large family. The team leader's personal characteristics influence the whole tone of this family and how it operates. The team leader must be able to tolerate ambiguity and the taking of judicious risks; otherwise, he or she will not be able to tolerate team members making important decisions independently, on the spot in the community, when the situation calls for it. This kind of action is absolutely necessary in the operation of an ACT program. To enhance the shared decision-making model, which is so important to the ACT team's operation, the team leader must be egalitarian by nature.

Likewise, if the team leader really believes in client participation, it is likely to happen. If the team leader is not easily frightened or easily made anxious, the whole team is more likely to handle crises in a calm and judicious manner. If the team leader is optimistic by nature and believes clients can improve, the optimism will be contagious and inspire the entire staff, as well as the clients. If the team leader is a mature person, it is much more likely that team interaction will also be mature and disputes based on personality differences will be diminished. If the team leader is energetic and enthusiastic, the whole team will mirror that temperament.

Working with this population is tough work and it is only human to rationalize behaviors that might make it a bit easier on staff but not be in the best interest of clients. It is up to the team leader to see that this does not happen; the team leader must always keep in mind that the goal of the team is to help clients and not make life easy for staff. In this regard, all team members, but especially the team leader, must act as a conscience for the team and remind each other, when necessary, that their first obligation is to the client. The team leader must believe that whatever needs to be done can be done. This attitude is contagious and will influence the whole team to have a "can do" attitude; thus, when a problem arises, time will be spent on how to solve it rather than on the reasons it can't be done.

As noted, this is very difficult work and staff are under a lot of pressure and need a great deal of support. The team leader must be sensitive to the team climate at all times and act when it needs attention. This may require having a special staff meeting or even a day-long retreat. In addition, the team leader must be aware of what is going on with individual staff members and provide the opportunity to ventilate and to receive support. It is a good idea for the team leader to have regularly scheduled half-hour individual meetings with staff members on a biweekly basis. It is wise for the team leader to be aware of the importance accorded to his or her assessments of other clinicians. The rule of thumb is to confront colleagues in private and praise them in public.

The personal characteristics of the team leader are vital, but so are his or her clinical skills. It is crucial that the team leader share in the clinical work and not just be an administrator. Sharing in the clinical work keeps the team leader in touch with the everyday problems of the clients and the everyday burdens carried by the staff. The team leader should spend at least 50 percent of his or her time doing the kind of clinical work done by the other staff members and, therefore, serve as the primary contact person for about six clients, half the normal caseload. Another function of the team leader, requiring excellent clinical skills, is the provision of clinical supervision to his or her staff members. The supervision is ordinarily carried out during the team meetings when the caseload is reviewed and client problems are being discussed and during treatment planning meetings, when treatment plans are being initially developed or updated. Generally, the first contact a client has with the team is a contact with the team leader. It is the team leader's responsibility to screen every potential new admission for appropriateness for the ACT team. What is required is a diagnosis of a major mental illness and sufficient functional disability to need the intense services, availability, and mobile outreach that the ACT team can provide.

The administrative duties of the team leader include chairing the hiring committee; collecting the data required by the parent organization or other funding sources; preparing budgets; performing annual performance reviews with his or her staff; handling questions and complaints from clients, family members, and other community members; resolving conflicts within the team; and being the interface between the ACT team and the parent organization, which is usually a mental health center. In addition, the team leader does a good bit of public relations work, making presentations to the community and other agencies.

The team leader is a middle management position, the most difficult of all administrative jobs. The team leader feels pressure from the parent organization—for example, to take more clients, to have staff prepare more reports, to have staff do more of the kinds of work that generate billable hours, etc. The team leader also feels pressure from the staff to resist such requests. The easy but not best solution is to resist the requests from the parent organization and ally yourself solely with the staff or to ignore the feelings of the staff and ally yourself solely with higher administration. The difficult but correct solution is to walk the thin line between staff and parent organization and to be seen by both as fair and reasonable. Doing this requires that the team leader keep the big picture in mind and never forget the long-term goal of the team; the big picture is to keep operating, so that the long-term goal of helping clients live a stable life of decent quality in the community can be achieved.

Suggested Readings

Dixon, L., Hackman, A., & Lehman, A. (in press). Consumer as staff in assertive community treatment programs. *Administration and Policy in Mental Health.*

Dixon, L. B., Krauss, N., Kerman, E., Lehman, A. F., & DeForge, B. R. (1995). Modifying the PACT model to serve homeless persons with severe mental illness. *Psychiatric Services, 46,* 684–688.

Dixon, L., Krauss, N., & Lehman, A. (1994). Consumers as providers: The promise and the challenge. *Community Mental Health Journal, 30,* 615–625.

Drake, R. E., & Osher, F. C. (1997). Treating substance abuse in patients with severe mental illness. In S. W. Henggeler & A. B. Santos (Eds.), *Innovative approaches for difficult-to-treat populations.* Washington: American Psychiatric Press.

Neale, M. S., & Rosenheck R. A. (1995). Theraputic alliance and outcome in a VA intensive case management program. *Psychiatric Services, 46,* 719–721.

Stein, L. I., & Test, M. A. (1976). Retraining hospital staff for work in a community program in Wisconsin. *Hospital & Community Psychiatry, 27,* 266–268.

··▶▶▶ 8 ◀◀◀··

Treatment Principles

Just as there are strategies to help the ACT team pace its services, there are treatment principles that guide its interventions. The preeminent principle that guides the team's actions can be stated in one sentence: The ACT team takes a broad approach to helping people with severe mental illnesses achieve a stable life of decent quality and will intervene in any domain to help achieve that goal. This chapter describes four domains of treatment principles: (1) structure and coordination of teamwork; (2) principles for working with the client; (3) principles for working with the community; and (4) principles for working with the family.

Structural Principles of Teamwork

Use a Team Approach to Accomplish Indicated Tasks

To ensure adequate continuous care and timely and effective episode-oriented care, the following tasks must be done:

1. Carefully evaluate the client to determine what skills and resources the ACT team must help the client acquire in order to achieve stability and a decent quality of life. Included here are such things as evaluation for psychotropic medication, a skills assessment for activities of daily living to determine where the client needs skill training, assessing housing needs, financial needs, etc.
2. Developing a comprehensive treatment plan to address the needs found in the evaluation.
3. Assuming responsibility for ensuring that all indicated services are provided; providing as many as possible directly and brokering the rest. It is of utmost importance to take responsibility for providing necessary services when brokered providers are not doing the job well.

4. Monitoring the client closely enough to change the treatment plan when needed.
5. Being able to intervene directly and/or cooperate with efforts at crisis stabilization whenever necessary.

Accomplishing the tasks noted above requires twenty-four-hour availability and expertise in several areas, e.g., clinical, rehabilitative, and practical help and support. Furthermore, the interrelatedness of all these interventions and supports cannot be overemphasized. Therefore, they must be provided in a way that ensures that they are integrated with one another and are timed to be relevant to the client's current situation.

The frequency of relapse back to the psychotic phase, as well as the duration and severity of the relapse, is closely related to how well the tasks described above are carried out. If these tasks are not done well, clients will experience frequent relapses and frequent hospitalizations and life between relapses will be experienced as chaotic and meaningless. If, on the other hand, these tasks are done well, their lives will be more stable, they will be more likely to have satisfying interpersonal relationships, they will more likely be involved in activities they feel are worthwhile, and they will, to a significantly greater degree, experience meaning in their lives. The complex set of tasks and responsibilities noted above cannot be accomplished by one professional discipline; it can only be achieved by a multidisciplinary team that has the expertise, sufficient staff, and time to carry out these tasks.

Share Responsibility

The responsibility for the total client caseload is shared by all, even though persons on the team serve as the primary contacts for their specified group of clients. In this model, over time, every team member gets to know every client and every client gets to know every team member. As will be described in the next chapter, one team member can be responsible for certain administrative tasks for a designated number of clients, but the clinical work and responsibility are shared by all team members. The next chapter will detail how the team operationalizes this principle.

Sharing responsibility among the team members yields advantages for both the clients and the staff. For the staff, utilizing this shared caseload approach has been very effective in preventing burnout—staff morale is high and turnover is quite low. Some staff work more with some clients than with others; this is based on staff-client "fit" rather than arbitrary assignment. The advantage is that those staff and clients who work well together do so, and staff and clients who don't get along so well tend to do less business with each other.

This model also has several advantages for the client: Since the client gets to know and work with many members of the team, the departure of one team member does not create a major problem for the client. This contrasts with the single case manager model, where the client relates primarily to one person and, since there is a notoriously high turnover rate, the client frequently has to deal with the loss of an important relationship and go through the process of developing a new one, with the knowledge that this new relationship will probably not last long either. The shared team approach has another advantage for clients, who vary in the degree to which they want or can use a close relationship with one person. This model allows for a variety of situations to best fit the client's needs. If it is helpful to the client to develop a strong one-to-one relationship, the team can accommodate that. If, on the other hand, it is best for the client not to do so, the team can provide many staff to work with that client.

It has already been noted that ACT team members have high morale and experience low turnover. This is because the team approach of sharing the caseload provides a number of benefits for the staff. One benefit is the opportunity to get respite when needed. Working with individuals with high needs is very stressful and there are times when a staff member may feel that he or she just cannot face a client that day and survive. With the team approach, that staff member can ask for, and receive, a day free of client contact. The staff member can spend the day on paperwork or making phone calls. Other staff members are willing to accommodate because they know that when they are having a similar day they will get the same consideration.

Another advantage is the opportunity for group celebration when something goes well. For example, if the team has been working hard to convince a client to get cleaned up so that he does not go around smelling badly and the client finally takes a bath and puts on fresh clothing, it is something to note and celebrate. When only one person has been trying to get that to happen and it finally does, it is hard to celebrate the event. With the team approach, however, all have been aware of the problem, many have worked on it, so the celebration is spontaneous and real when it happens.

Sharing grief is a tremendous advantage offered by the team approach. You can't work with this population without negative events occurring. Clients relapse and become psychotic and, since the rate of suicide in persons with schizophrenia is quite high, suicides do occur. These are terrible burdens to carry. Having a team to share both the grief and the responsibility makes an enormous difference in one's work life.

Share Governance

Since the team utilizes a shared caseload model, the question of how decisions are made regarding clients is a crucial one. We believe that these teams work best when the decisions are made under a shared governance model. Shared governance, in turn, works best when there is an agreed-upon ground rule that decisions grow from value-based discussions (the team spends time identifying and "signing on" core values that guide decisions and actions).

As will be described in the next chapter, the team meets on a daily basis to review clients, discuss problems, and make decisions about what needs to be done. Although the team leader leads the discussion, all team members are expected to be involved in the discourse and to make any comments and recommendations they feel may be useful. When there are differences of opinion, the discussion continues until there is a general consensus on the approach to be taken. For example, in the case of a client who had not been budgeting his money very well and is receiving daily allotments from the team, the time will come to return more control to him. When that time should be and whether the allotments should be changed so that they are given once every three days or once a week are important questions. With the ACT team model, everyone knows the client and it is expected that the decision will be a team decision, not one made by a single person on the team. It is unacceptable for a team member to relinquish responsibility for the decision to someone else. Certainly, everyone cannot be totally comfortable with every decision made; with shared governance, it is often necessary to go along with a decision one is not totally comfortable with. The question one must ask of oneself is, "Is this decision one that may have serious negative consequences for the client?" If not, then the staff member must learn to live with a decision he or she does not fully agree with. However, if the team member thinks the pending decision will have serious negative consequences, it is his or her responsibility to keep the discussion going until a more satisfactory decision is reached. With this shared governance model, some team members' input may be given more weight than that of other team members. This is usually based on who knows the client best, who might have special expertise in that particular area, and, very importantly, who, over time, has proven him- or herself to be highly competent. Influence on the team is not obtained by the letters after one's name; it is earned through demonstrated competence.

It may seem that the above-described process would be very time-consuming and inefficient; it does take time, but it is highly efficient. It is efficient because it utilizes the collective knowledge and wisdom of everyone on the team and all feel that what they do makes a real difference in what and how decisions are made. This last point cannot be overemphasized. Members of the team spend a great deal of time in the field working independently with clients. When staff know that what they do and think is taken seriously, this gives them the motivation to work hard and make decisions, even difficult ones, on the spot when it is clear that something needs to be done immediately. This is reinforced by another important principle of ACT: "When in doubt, do something." At the next team meeting, what was done is discussed. Staff are never criticized for what they did. There will often be a discussion as to how it might be done differently the next time it comes up; however, the team member will always by praised for doing what he or she did, rather than waiting.

Cross-train Team Members

The ACT team is multidisciplinary, with team members having special expertise in various areas. An important principle is that full advantage is taken of each team member's expertise, but that expertise is not the sole property of that team member. The principle is further employed by making it the responsibility of staff with special expertise to teach as much as is feasible to the other team members. Thus, in the ACT team, team members cross-train one another so that all have some familiarity with the functions of their colleagues. For example, a psychiatric paraprofessional learns to recognize medication side effects so that he or she can alert the psychiatrist as soon as the side effects are perceived; psychiatrists learn about agencies and will interact with an agency that insists on talking to "the doctor."

Integrate Services

ACT teams are best conceptualized as continuous care teams, that is, vehicles to provide whatever service or practical need a client requires. Services to address these needs fall into three broad categories: treatment, rehabilitation, and case management. By being the provider of most of these services (brokering for only a few), the continuous care team assures that the services are integrated and provided in the context of the client's current needs, with all activities directed toward helping the client make a stable life of decent quality in the community. Unfortunately, a high percentage of people with serious and persistent mental illness also suffer from substance abuse. This dually diagnosed group is best served when the substance abuse problem and the mental health problem are both addressed by the ACT team, rather than having another agency deal with the drug problem. This same principle holds true for rehabilitation. A safe generalization is, whatever the intervention, it will be more effective if it can be provided as an integrated part of the entire ACT program. Rehabilitation and drug abuse interventions will both be covered in detail later in the book.

Principles for Working with the Client

Enabling clients with serious and persistent mental illness to live successfully in the community requires helping not only the client but also members of the community. The next two sections will outline those two sets of principles. In the next chapter, describing the day-to-day operation of the ACT program, some of these principles will be illustrated by example.

Use an Assertive Approach

ACT is characterized by determined and positive action to achieve the basic goal of helping clients live successfully in the community. This principle infers acting quickly to avert negative consequences for clients, which, of course, requires careful client monitoring. Some have misconstrued the assertiveness of ACT to mean that the team acts aggressively to keep clients "under control." In fact, the assertive approach is directed toward shaping team member behavior rather than controlling clients. It dictates that the team must be assertive about knowing what is going on with clients and acting quickly and decisively when action is called for. ACT continually does what it can to increase client independence. The major goal of ACT is to help clients live successfully in the community, and the beauty of living in the community, as contrasted with living in an institution, is that clients are in control of their own lives.

Do a Careful Clinical Assessment

Virtually all of ACT's clients are persons with serious and persistent mental illness. In addition to doing a comprehensive clinical assessment of the client, the team obtains a careful history of prior treatments. This includes past hospitalizations, as well as past and current medications, their usefulness and their side effects. It is also useful to get a history of other psychiatric and/or psychological interventions and their effects. It is critically important to learn the client's feelings about and attitudes toward all of these treatments and his/her preferences.

Capitalize on Client Strengths

Traditional treatment programs focus primarily on pathology and pay little attention to the client's strengths. Rehabilitation programs, on the other hand, take advantage of strengths in designing the client's rehabilitation plan. Ordinarily, rehabilitation programs do not address pathology, leaving that task to those providing treatment for the client. The ACT model sees treatment and rehabilitation as highly interactive and believes that both are best accomplished when they are integrated and provided by the same entity; thus, in addition to carefully evaluating the client's pathology and designing a clinical intervention for treating it, the team evaluates the client's strengths and utilizes them in designing a rehabilitation plan.

Tailor Programming to Individual Needs

After each client's needs are comprehensively evaluated, a treatment and rehabilitation program is designed, in concert with the client, specifically to meet that client's needs and wishes; the plan is updated periodically. Through this process, programming is highly individualized. This contrasts with programs that routinely involve clients in standard ongoing treatments, where, for example, everyone is in group therapy or in a medication clinic.

Deliver Services In Vivo

To effectively adhere to the basic principle, many services must be provided in the community. For example, if a client needs help getting his apartment cleaned and will face eviction if that is not done, it is imperative that this be accomplished. Talking to the client in an office or trying to teach him how to clean his apartment in a day treatment setting is not likely to work nearly as well as having someone go to his apartment, show him what needs to be done, and, if necessary, help him do it. This same in vivo approach is necessary in a myriad of situations, from accompanying a frightened client to the dentist to working with the client and family members in their home. The bottom line is always the same—whatever needs to be done must be done and done well; this often requires that the task be done in vivo, out in the community.

Titrate Support

As interdependent human beings we all need support to withstand the daily trials and tribulations of life. Most people have a family, jobs, and friends to help cushion the stresses of everyday life. However, life for persons with serious and persistent mental illness is especially difficult. Most live at the poverty level and have significant disabilities. Compounding the problem is the fact that most do not have highly satisfying jobs and many have tenuous interpersonal relationships and so spend a lot of time alone. Our clients need a great deal of support just to keep going. Many mental health professionals were taught that giving support was not a good thing. That may be true if one is psychoanalyzing a well functioning person; however, for persons with serious and persistent mental illness, sufficient support is crucial. Certainly, giving too much support is not good either; a good rule to follow is: When in doubt as to whether to give support or not, give it. The authors have been working with persons with serious and persistent mental illness for many years and we can honestly say that some of the most courageous people we have known are persons with serious and persistent mental illness who, despite great adversity and obstacles, struggle every day to make a life for themselves in the community.

Relate to Clients as Responsible Citizens

It is imperative to accept—and believe it to the core of one's soul—that ACT clients are first and foremost citizens, with all the rights and responsibilities of citizenship, and secondarily that they happen to be citizens who have a serious and persistent mental illness. Believing this is crucial when working with clients or with other community members and agencies. As citizens, ACT clients have a right to live in the community and to benefit from any and all services available to other citizens in the community. An important part of an ACT staff member's job is to advocate for the rights of ACT clients. Persons with serious and persistent mental illness are among the most discriminated against groups in society, and the struggle to help them live successfully in the community is as much a civil rights issue as a clinical one.

Make Crisis Stabilization Services Available Twenty-Four Hours a Day

In helping a person with serious and persistent mental illness achieve long tenure in the community, it is essential that crises be dealt with promptly and effectively. Conceptually, it is important to differentiate between crisis intervention and crisis stabilization. Most crisis units in the United States, the majority of which are located in the emergency room of a hospital, do crisis intervention, which consists of doing an evaluation and making a disposition. Typically, an individual mental health worker evaluates the case and decides, after the initial contact, if the person requires hospitalization or can wait to be seen by the outpatient department, where it is not unusual for there to be a waiting list. Other alternatives, such as stabilizing the crisis through a home visit or putting the person in a crisis bed, are ordinarily not available. Since whether a person is hospitalized depends on the interaction between that individual's problem and the services that are immediately available in the community to manage the problem, it is clear that the more services immediately available for the client, the less need for hospitalization. As a result, when all that can be done is evaluation and disposition, many people are hospitalized who could be managed quite easily in the community if, instead, they had received a crisis stabilization approach.

In crisis stabilization, a careful evaluation is done with the primary goal of stabilizing the crisis, not merely making a dispositional recommendation. The ACT team does crisis stabilization. The client in crisis is evaluated in the setting most likely to provide the information needed to develop the stabilization plan, whether that be the client's home, the police station, etc. Then the client is seen as often as necessary, which may be several times a day for several days. In addition, when necessary, others are involved who may be useful in stabilizing the crisis, such as family, significant others, employers, etc.

Most ACT teams have a rotating call schedule, whereby one of the staff is on call to respond to crisis situations. Many crises can be managed by phone; for those that cannot it is imperative that the staff member meet with the client face-to-face. In other situations, ACT teams are part of a mental health center and collaborate with the crisis unit of their center to manage the crises of their clients when they occur after the ACT evening shift. For that to work successfully, several conditions must be met: The crisis unit of the center must truly be an effective crisis stabilization unit; like the ACT team itself, the crisis unit needs to be mobile and able to go to the client when necessary. The staffs of the ACT team and the crisis unit must have a close working relationship. The ACT staff must be willing to be called at night by the crisis team to give information about any client of theirs that the crisis team has contact with and needs information about. For clients that have frequent and similar crises, the ACT team should prepare a crisis plan outlining the management of the crisis and the center's crisis unit should have a copy of that plan on file. It is important to emphasize that the center's crisis team does not take over the crisis; it collaborates with the ACT team when the ACT staff are off duty.

Principles for Work with the Community

Providing support to the community members who are in contact with ACT clients, including family members, landlords, storekeepers, employers, and community agencies, is just as important as working with the clients themselves. These community members' attitudes towards clients and modes of relating to them are significant factors in influencing how well the clients do. The following are the principles used in working with the community.

Use an Assertive Approach

Just as appropriate assertiveness is crucial in working with clients, it is also crucial in working with the community. For example, if one lets things slide with a landlord or an agency to the point where the decision has been made to evict or terminate the client, it is then usually too late to repair the problem. The client has lost a resource, and the results of this loss not only are stressful to the client but also create a great deal of work for the staff. The team must closely monitor the relationship that the client has with the community and intervene early if difficulty arises.

Use a Wide Variety of Community Resources

There are many public agencies that advertise themselves as providing services to the citizens of the community, but never anticipate that they might be asked to provide those services to psychiatric clients. Always remember, the client is first and foremost a citizen and, as such, is entitled to any services available to citizens. Thus, we recommend making use of any agency in the community that can be of value to the client. The agency will, in all probability, initially require education and support from the ACT team. We cannot emphasize too strongly that agency cooperation is not obtained by simply demanding it. Staff must provide sufficient support and education to those agencies in order to gain their cooperation.

As an example, until a few years ago the Visiting Nurse Service (VNS) of Dane County, Wisconsin, had virtually no psychiatric clients on its caseload. Now these nurses are working with a number of psychiatric clients with medical needs; they change dressings, provide help to clients with diabetes, etc., and in so doing provide support to clients in their homes. In addition, they serve as an additional resource to monitor client functioning. Thus, the VNS has become a valuable asset to the Dane County mental health system. When VNS was first approached, they were not jubilant about the thought of doing what they are now quite happy to do. They said, "We really don't know much about treating psychiatric clients and will probably do them more harm than good. Our staff does not have proper training." Clearly their anxiety was overdetermined. They needed support, education, and reassurance. They were told that an ACT staff member would accompany their staff member until their staff felt comfortable without the presence of an ACT team member coming along with them. Further, they were told that once they got to know the client as a person, they would feel comfortable working with him or her and do a competent job. They agreed and were given the support and on-the-job training they needed. Within a short time they were comfortable enough to serve clients without the presence of an ACT staff person. An added bonus is that the VNS has become a strong advocate for community treatment. The ACT team has had the same experience with other agencies that have not had experience with seriously mentally ill people. Once they get to know the clients and work with them over a period of time, prejudices or myths that they might have had evaporate.

Not all community agencies are this responsive. To make sure that individuals with a mental illness are granted the same rights and access to community resources as other citizens, the U.S. Congress passed the Americans with Disabilities Act. Under Title I of the ADA, the first avenue of recourse for individuals with disabilities who feel they have been discriminated against is the filing of a charge of employment discrimination with the U.S. Equal Employment Opportunity Commission (EEOC). Public funding mechanisms such as United Way or the U.S. Public Health Service specifically prohibit discrimination based on disability.

If one is truly interested in getting the community to work with and accept persons with severe and persistent mental illness, one may have to press very hard, to be assertive and even "pushy." It is difficult for staff to do this unless they truly believe that their clients have a right to these services, a right to live in the community, and do not have to feel humbly grateful to the rest of the community for allowing their clients to be there. Ideally, staff should feel this to the depth of their souls, so that they can imbue and instill these values in both their clients and in the other members of the community. However, let us emphasize again that agency cooperation is not obtained by simply demanding it; staff must provide sufficient support and education to those agencies in order to gain their cooperation.

Provide Support and Education to Community Members

In order to gain community acceptance and cooperation, it is vital to provide support and education to families, landlords, shopkeepers, employers, and anyone else with whom clients have significant contact. Rather than attempting to mount a mass education program for the community, we recommend that the ACT team educate and support community members every time a problem arises between a client and a community member. For example, if a client were having trouble with a shopkeeper, we would suggest getting together with the shopkeeper and the client with several goals in mind: first, with the client present, teaching the shopkeeper how to relate to the client in a very straightforward and unambiguous manner; then, to use the event as an opportunity to teach about serious mental illness and help the shopkeeper understand why a community-based approach is far better than institutional care. It is also useful to give a civics lesson by emphasizing that, although we might not approve of how some people dress or act, as good citizens we must be willing to tolerate deviant behaviors that are not against the law. Finally, we would leave the shopkeeper a card with the ACT team's phone number on it and urge him or her to call anytime, twenty-four hours a day, seven days a week, if he or she experiences any problems or has questions relating to the client. Although some problems may remain, providing this kind of education and support will help clients gain greater community acceptance.

Retain Responsibility for Client Care

People with serious mental illness require an array of different services; although the ACT team will provide the bulk of the services, some will be provided by other agencies, running the gamut from the county welfare agency to a medical clinic for physical health care. The interrelatedness of all these interventions and supports cannot be overemphasized. They must be provided in a way that ensures that they are integrated with one another and are timed to be relevant to the client's current situation. It is the ACT team's responsibility to see that good coordination among all these agencies is accomplished. In the past, mental health practitioners have relied on traditional referral and on interagency communication to attain coordinated and continuous services for clients. Unfortunately, this has not worked well. Too often, services have been poorly coordinated, incomplete, and porous—clients have "fallen through the cracks." Although referral and interagency communication are necessary, they are not sufficient. The keystone to coordinated and continuous services is having a fixed point of responsibility for client care. Even though there are many agencies providing services, one agency, the ACT team, must remain responsible to see that all the services are delivered.

Since all programs have clients that tax their limits, at some point an agency working with an ACT client may terminate their work with the client. The ACT program, in addition to ensuring coordination, must retain responsibility for the care that client was getting from the terminating agency. To do this, it must provide that care until the client is well connected with another agency. If another program cannot be found, the ACT team must continue to work with the client. Retaining responsibility also means recognizing that many ACT clients have lifelong disorders; thus, a commitment must be made for as long as the client needs help, which may be for the rest of his or her life. The amount of service given during that lifetime varies tremendously. Some clients do so well that all they need is a telephone call once a month to find out how they are doing. Other clients require daily contact in their home. For most clients, the amount of input varies over time. To operate as efficiently as possible, we give clients just what they need, when they need it and where they need it. In summary, retaining responsibility is crucial; it means providing most of the services within the ACT program and ensuring that there is good agency coordination for services provided elsewhere and that treatment continues for as long as the client requires it.

Principles for Working with the Families

Family members and the ACT team members become something of a task force, in which experts from various sectors of the patient's total network share experiences, information, planning, and the creation of new ideas and options, especially in the difficult area of vocational rehabilitation. The professional team's job is then to take these possibilities and attempt to realize them.

—Bill McFarlane

For too long the families of our clients have carried a double burden: the burden of having a member of their family stricken with a severe and disabling illness; and that of hearing mental health professionals say that they were responsible for that illness, that the mother was schizophrenogenic, or that the husband-wife relationship was pathological and caused a schizophrenic child, or that the whole family was sick and that the "identified client" was carrying everyone's pathology so that the rest of them could appear well. These theories were very seductive and, unfortunately, influenced at least three generations of mental health professionals. They are, however, post hoc theories supported by very little data. There are ample data that support the predominant role of biological factors in the etiology of schizophrenia and bipolar disorders. We help neither the client nor the client's family nor the field by making anyone feel guilty or responsible for the illness. Working effectively with the client often requires the cooperation of the family. Understandably, a family feeling wrongly accused and so hostile towards the treaters is unlikely to cooperate. Often it is useful for the client and the family to have the client move to a higher level of independence by moving away from his family's home—a process termed "constructive separation." This may be difficult in any case; it is almost impossible if the family is made to feel guilty. Whether clients are separated from their families or not, the ACT team continues to work closely with the family, using problem-solving, psychoeducational approaches.

Family psychoeducation is a group of clearly articulated principles designed to inform families about the state of knowledge on mental illnesses, create a home environment that minimizes relapse-induced stress, and create convalescent environments that can facilitate recuperation from illness episodes. The basic assumptions about the nature of severe mental illness that are presented to families as operational principles to be used by staff and family members in the process of problem solving are as follows:

- Severe mental illnessess have clear and demonstrable causative biological components.
- Severe mental illnesses are lifelong conditions characterized by episodes of symptom intensity, which can diminish slowly in the absence of stress.
- One of the impairments resulting from severe mental illness involves attention and arousal, such that a person's ability to gate stimuli adequately is impaired.
- Families can have an influence on this biological process so that they are either able to protect the individual from episodes of symptom intensity or appear to inadvertently exacerbate them.
- Living with a mentally ill relative has consequences for the family, in that the stigma associated with the illness negatively impacts on the social support networks of the family.

Recently, Robert McFarlane and his colleagues have integrated family psychoeducation into the framework of ACT. The merging of family psychoeducation into ACT programs fosters the maximum possible coordination between all the important people and social forces in an individual's life. In this fashion, the families become close collaborators in developing the treatment and rehabilitation plan. The professional team's job is then to take these possibilities and attempt to realize them.

When family psychoeducation is provided to several families at a time, the approach also serves to counter family isolation and stigma. Families are encouraged to expand their social networks by participating in group problem-solving, supporting one another, and socializing outside of the group. The multiple-family format is an ideal way for family members to learn from each other about situations that are likely to be stressful for their relatives and about ways to assist them in overcoming obstacles. Additionally, the family rebuilds its network of family and friends, which has usually been weakened as a consequence of the illness. There is a real sense of working towards a common goal in the structured multiple-family format, as individual client's goals are formulated by the whole group as part of the multiple-family group meetings.

Suggested Readings

Falloon, I. R. H., & Liberman, R. P. (1983). Behavioral family interventions in the management of chronic schizophrenia. In W. R. McFarlane (Ed.), *Family therapy in schizophrenia*. New York: Guilford.

McFarlane, W. R. (1997). Family psychoeducation: Basic concepts and innovative applications. In S. W. Henggeler & A. B. Santos (Eds.), *Innovative approaches for difficult-to-treat populations*. Washington: American Psychiatric Press.

McFarlane, W. R. (1997). Integrating family psychoeducation and assertive community treatment. *The Journal of Mental Health Administration and Policy Special Issue on Assertive Community Treatment*.

Stein, L. I. (1992, Fall). On the abolishment of the case manager. *Health Affairs*, 172–177.

Stein, L. I. (1992). Crisis stabilization services for persons with psychotic illnesses. In J. B. van Luyn, et al. (Eds.), *Emergency psychiatry today* (pp. 25-28). New York: Elsevier Science.

··›♪➋ 9 ❨❨❨··

Daily Program Operation

This chapter describes how an ACT program operates in order to help mentally ill persons achieve stability, enjoy a decent quality of life, and move toward recovery. It is intended as the book's "nuts and bolts" section to describe and give guidance in the day-to-day operation of an ACT program. In organizing this chapter, we struggled with what should come first—staff activities (staff meetings, treatment plan development, etc.) or the overall framework within which the staff operates (hours of operation, layout of the office space, etc.). There are advantages and disadvantages to either approach; however, we felt that providing a framework first had the merit of furnishing a structural context for the content on staff activities.

The Physical Layout

Over time, all staff members will interact to some extent with every person on the team's caseload. In addition, during staff meetings, when decisions need to be made regarding individual clients, virtually all staff will be involved in the discussion. Clearly, the more knowledgeable staff are about all the program's clients, the better able they are to work with them and contribute intelligently during staff discussions. The layout of the ACT program's space is designed to facilitate communication between staff members and thus enhance their knowledge of all persons assigned to their care. Critical to this process is a room spacious enough to hold a large table, around which all staff members can comfortably sit. Staff meetings are held at this table. Virtually every ACT program we know has a space with a large table.

Another aspect of space that all programs have in common is a medication room. This room can be locked and has a medication cabinet that can also be locked. It is very useful for this room to also have a wash basin. The medication room is used to store medications, give injections, and sort and package medications for those programs that do not have a pharmacy to do that task.

Except for these two mandatory rooms, ACT programs around the country have varied layouts. One important variable is the degree to which the ACT team members have individual offices. We recommend having very few, if any, individual offices. In their place, we suggest that the staff meeting room be a very large room, with the meeting table in the center and staff members' desks located around the periphery of the room. Thus, when staff members are not in the community and are back "at the office," they will be working out in the open where easy and free communication between staff members is almost unavoidable. In many ACT programs this large open space has been termed the "bull pen." Certainly, private space is mandatory for certain activities, from individual counseling sessions to family work. To accommodate that need, the ACT program needs private office spaces of various sizes, which are available to everyone. This, of course, requires signing up in advance whenever possible. For emergent situations, when a private space is unavailable, the ACT team does what it always does—it gets the job done as best as possible given whatever limitations are imposed on it at the time. For example, a client or family member might be invited to go for a walk to attain privacy, or staff may be asked to vacate their space temporarily, etc. Limitations are never used as an excuse for not doing whatever must be done.

The entry area, usually the area that immediately precedes the bull pen, is the secretary's area, which also acts as a small waiting room. As described in an earlier section, the secretary is the interface between the staff and the clients, as well as between the staff and the rest of the community. This space must be an inviting environment and reflect the variety of cultures and lifestyles of the community. Clients must come to feel that the ACT program is really there for them, cares about them, and, when necessary, will fight for them. Their waiting room, and how they are related to when they are in it, must convey that message.

One more word about space. It is very useful to have on the wall large "blackboards," which can be updated daily and referred to during staff meetings. Examples include a board that has clients' names and pressing issues which must be discussed at that day's staff meeting; a board that has the name of each person who is hospitalized, showing the date of hospitalization, as well as the names of ACT and hospital personnel working with the hospitalized patient; and a board showing clients who are employed.

Hours of Operation

The ACT team will be available every day of the year, including holidays, to provide treatment, rehabilitation, and support activities. It also has the capability of responding to crises twenty-four hours a day. How an ACT team fulfills that requirement varies from place to place, depending on the availability of other services. For example, when the parent organization has a well functioning crisis resolution team that works collaboratively with the ACT program, it can be used to collaborate with the ACT team in responding to crises when the team is off duty. In any case, the program should operate a minimum of twelve hours a day on weekdays and eight hours a day on weekends and holidays. On weekdays, shifts should be arranged so that the peak hours of operation, usually from 10:30 A.M. to 4:30 P.M., are the most heavily staffed. Whether shifts are rotated or kept constant varies from place to place; however, we recommend rotating both evening and weekend shifts, if possible.

During program off-hours, a member of the staff rotates to take on-call duty and respond to crisis calls. While most of these can be managed by phone, the staff member must be prepared to go out to where the crisis is occurring. All staff should be willing to respond to telephone calls from the staff person on call or the crisis unit to give information about a person who is in a crisis situation.

Having a psychiatrist available during all off-hours is enormously helpful. How this is done varies from site to site. Some ACT psychiatrists are willing to take calls when not on duty; at other sites an alternative is utilized, such as using the psychiatrist on-call at the mental health center or the hospital emergency room.

An Emergency Fund

An emergency fund for ACT clients is very useful and should be budgeted for at a level of around $2,000 per 100 ACT clients. These monies are often used for purchasing necessary extra health care products or medications. At times this fund may determine whether a person will obtain decent housing. For example, renting an apartment usually requires a security deposit and one month's rent in advance. Many clients don't have that much money in reserve. A person in this situation can take a loan from the emergency fund and pay it back on a reasonable repayment schedule set up by the team. Other uses of the fund include a loan to pay the rent if it comes due while the person is in the hospital, a loan to tide them over in times of financial need, etc. The great majority of the fund is given out in loans and so the fund regenerates itself for the most part. Each year, the fund needs only a small amount of money to bring it up to the original amount. Therefore, for a relatively small initial outlay, a great deal of benefit may accrue.

The Referral and Admissions Process

Potential referral sources, agencies, and service providers are given a description of the ACT program, an explanation of how this service fits into the system of care, and a description of the kinds of individuals it is best fitted to serve. Part of this information is a list of the specific criteria required for admission into the program. When a referral is obtained, the team leader gathers information from various sources to determine if the referral does, indeed, meet the admission requirements. When individuals fit admission criteria, further information is collected to facilitate the first meeting with them.

The ACT program must have specified admission criteria to ensure that the caseload selected requires the staff intensity and availability that an ACT program can provide. An all too common problem in the United States is that the clients who are difficult to work with often get neglected and, as a result, do very poorly. This is not only unfortunate for those individuals but also detrimental to the entire treatment system. Because of the lack of appropriate community treatment, these folks require a great deal of expensive hospital care and consume an inordinate proportion of the available mental health budget, which leaves insufficient funds for the development of a comprehensive system of care for all the people in the system. Appropriate admission criteria protect both the system and the service users by ensuring that those in greatest need of an ACT program are the ones who are actually admitted to the program. The following admission criteria are adapted from those used by ACT units of the Dane County Mental Health Center, Inc.:

1. Individuals with a primary diagnosis of schizophrenia, schizoaffective disorder, or severe affective disorder who have had several psychotic episodes and psychiatric hospitalizations are given the highest priority for admission.

2. Other eligible individuals are those who have a major mental disorder, who by history or prognosis are likely to require intermittent acute intensive or prolonged intensive care (i.e., hospital inpatient or nursing home care), or are likely to live in a severely dysfunctional manner if ACT services are not provided, and who exhibit persistent disability or impairment in major areas of community living as evidenced by:

   a. vocational impairment manifested by an inability to be consistently employed at a self-sustaining level, an ability to be employed only with extensive supports, or recurrent unemployment because of psychotic episodes, despite ability to earn sustaining income.

b. educational impairment manifested by an inability to establish and pursue educational goals within a normal time frame without extensive supports.

c. impairment in homemaker functioning, as shown by an inability to consistently and independently carry out home management tasks, including preparing meals, washing clothes, budgeting, completing child-care tasks and responsibilities. When part-time homemaker and educational or vocational roles coexist, the functional level of the combined roles are assessed according to existing community norms.

d. impairment in social or interpersonal functioning manifested by a person's inability to independently develop or maintain adult social relationships or to independently participate in adult social or recreational activities. Such impairment is evidenced by repeated inappropriate or inadequate social behavior, or the ability to behave appropriately only with extensive support and coaching, or involvement that is mostly limited to special activities established for others with impairments.

e. impairment in community functioning as shown by a pattern of significant community disruptions that may not occur often but are of such magnitude that they result in consequences such as exclusion, incarceration, or impediments to securing basic needs such as housing.

f. impairments in self-care or independent living manifested by a person's inability to consistently perform, without significant support and assistance, a range of practical daily living tasks, including grooming, hygiene, clothes washing, meeting nutritional needs, care of personal business affairs, transportation, care of residence, procurement of medical, legal, and housing services, recognition and avoidance of common dangers and hazards to self and possessions.

3. Individuals with a singular principal diagnosis of chemical abuse, organic brain syndrome, developmental disability, or personality disorder are not eligible. However, if a person has a primary diagnosis of a major mental illness and any of the above conditions as a secondary diagnosis, he or she will be eligible for ACT services.

The First Meeting with the Client

Prior to the first meeting it is useful to have sufficient information to help guide the interaction, as well as to inspire credibility by demonstrating that a good bit of work and thought has already been done prior to the meeting. The following information should be obtained prior to the first meeting:

1. Name, address, sex, date of birth.
2. Primary diagnosis and previous diagnoses.
3. Marital/family status and living situation.
4. Suicide/homicide potential as assessed by referral source.
5. Medications, current and past, and degree of compliance.
6. Legal status, conditional release, probation, parole, etc.
7. Involvement with other agencies and services, current and past.
8. Current therapist and psychiatrist.
9. Recommendations from the referral source as to services anticipated to be needed from the ACT team.
10. Other information that might be useful in choosing the team member who will serve as the primary contact person.

Mentally ill persons referred to ACT programs are often resistant to treatment, so the approach used at the very first meeting must be one that will be experienced as welcoming and nonthreatening. Keep in mind that in many cases the individual's past experiences with the mental health system have involved a loss of control and so the issue of control is often a major one. In the first meeting it must be made clear that the client will be an active participant in all decisions regarding his or her care. A good way to start is to learn from the client where the first meeting should take place; that is, would he or she prefer to come to where the program is located or a different location?

The team leader is the staff person who first meets with the new client. In some ACT programs, the primary contact person also attends. The choice of primary contact person is based on information obtained prior to the first meeting. For example, if during the preadmission data-gathering it was learned that the individual tends to feel competitive with males and does much better relating to females, a woman staff member would be chosen to be his primary contact person (if it becomes clear, over time, that this choice does not lead to a good fit between the client and primary contact person, another primary contact person would be chosen). After introductions and a brief description of the program, the first meeting should focus on two major tasks: (a) to be responsive to questions about the program; (b) to ensure that sometime during the meeting (unless an emergency situation exists) the client gets the following information:

1. The general nature and purpose of the ACT program.
2. The hours during which services are routinely available.

3. Service costs and who will be billed.
4. His or her rights and the grievance procedure available to him or her if he or she is dissatisfied with the program.
5. Program rules governing his or her conduct and the consequences of infractions of those rules and, importantly, the process available to him or her for review and appeal.
6. The program's procedures for follow-up if a client is discharged.

At the conclusion of the first meeting, a mutually acceptable time and place for the next contact with the client will be established. The client is then informed that, within a short time, he or she will be involved with the staff in completing an in-depth assessment, historical review, and the development of the initial treatment plan.

The Development of the Initial Treatment Plan

The first step in developing the treatment plan, whether it is the initial plan, the comprehensive plan, or the six-month follow-up plan, is careful assessment. Assessment, the most critical element of the ACT approach, is a continuous activity, achieved through conscientious monitoring, and is the basis for guiding staff interventions.

The initial assessment is completed as soon as possible after admission to the program. Usually, enough information is obtained after the first visit to do so (see appendix for Initial Assessment and Plan). It is done with the participation of the client to the greatest degree possible (there are times when the person is not yet willing to participate; at those times, it is done without their contribution). The initial assessment includes psychiatric diagnoses, current medications, housing situation, financial situation, and preliminary information on functional impairment, if any, in the following areas: vocational, educational, homemaking, social/interpersonal, community integration, and activity of daily living (ADL) skills. The primary purpose of the initial assessment is to quickly develop an immediate initial treatment plan to ensure that pressing needs are addressed and begin to work on long-range goals; these will be more fully developed within thirty days in the first comprehensive treatment plan.

The In-depth Assessment

Immediately following the implementation of the initial treatment plan, the primary contact person's responsibility is to see to it that the information needed to develop a comprehensive treatment plan is collected. This plan is the foundation for guiding the team's long-term work with the client. The appendix has a series of assessment forms that are used by the Mental Health Center of Dane County, Inc. (MHCDC) to record various areas of information needed for the chart and to write the comprehensive treatment plan. The completed forms do not constitute the treatment plan but are used as a tool to write the plan, which is in narrative form. The client should be involved as much as possible in the development of the plan, which should be completed within a month after admission to the program. The comprehensive treatment plan is to be updated in writing at least once every six months.

Following is a brief summary of the assessment material to be collected and used in the development of the comprehensive treatment plan. There are fifteen domains in which information is collected. Forms developed by MHCDC for each of those domains are located in the appendix. Information for the first twelve forms is obtained from the client; the last three forms—agency, family and significant-other interviews—are completed only with the client's consent. To give the reader an idea of the kind of material found on the forms, the domains are listed below, with a sampling of some of the categories found on the forms.

1. *Psychiatric Functioning and History.* Current medications and dosage; medication compliance (specifics on whether medication is delivered, taken independently, etc.); what side effects does the client report; what side effects did the examiner note; what preferences for medication does client have; attendance at psychiatric appointments—willingly, regularly, etc.; has client received education regarding his or her mental illness and medications; what is the client's understanding of the illness; how does the mental illness make the client feel; perception of the treatment and support received—what seemed to help and what didn't; how do symptoms interfere with daily functioning—specify which symptom affects which area of functioning; a complete mental status examination.

2. *Psychiatric Hospitalization.* A record of psychiatric hospitalizations.

3. *Health History.* Name of the client's primary care physician, dentist, eye doctor; occupational health—physical conditions which may affect employment, injuries sustained at work, etc.; nutritional information—typical daily food intake; sleeping habits; health history—adult and childhood; immunizations; sex-related topics—birth control, sexually transmitted diseases; family health history; current health status.

4. *Alcohol and Drug Assessment.* Client's report of drug usage; view of family and friends regarding client's drug usage (as reported by client); negative events in client's life related to drug use; family history of drug use.

5. ***Activities of Daily Living.*** Food and nutrition skills, in addition to availability of cooking facilities and refrigeration; typical day's diet; an evaluation of maintenance and housekeeping skills; personal hygiene and grooming skills; transportation use—bus, cab, bike, etc.; recreation and leisure skills; social skills; interpersonal skills; money management skills.

6. ***Culturological History.*** Learning about the client's culture and ethnicity; discussion of cultural differences between client and staff; learning about the client's religious/spiritual beliefs and values; learning about the client's culture, specifically, its explanations of mental illness and its beliefs about treatment; learning about the problems that stem from racism or discrimination.

7. ***Assessment of Family/Personal Relationships.*** Current relationships; parents' names and ages; siblings' names and ages; client's view of his or her relationship with all of the above.

8. ***Assessment of Informal/Formal Supports.*** Friends; family; whom client contacts when having a difficult time or when wanting to share something happy; church; twelve-step programs; clubs and organizations; agencies, including primary contact for each agency.

9. ***Financial Information.*** Benefits—SSI, SSDI, VA benefits, earnings, food stamps, other benefits; description of current monthly budget—rent, utilities, food, etc.

10. ***Residential History.*** Living situations since childhood; current address and telephone number; condition of living situation; getting along with landlord and neighbors; current living companions.

11. ***Vocational Profile.*** Job preference; disabilities that may interfere with work; financial or medical benefits that may be disincentives to work; availability of transportation; endurance level regarding ability to work (number of hours per day); work history, including type of job, hours per week, relationship with employer and co-workers, etc.; work skills; time awareness; motivation to work; effect of work on symptoms.

12. ***Assessment of Legal Involvement.*** History of involuntary hospitalizations; does client have a guardian or representative payee—if so, name, address, and phone number; history of arrest and incarceration; history of parole and probation; other legal involvement—eviction, suits, etc.

13. ***Agency Interviews.*** Name of agency and primary contact person; service provided; degree of client involvement with the agency; agency's assessment of client's strengths and weaknesses; agency and client goals in agency program; agency's opinion as to how ACT could assist client; agency's suggestion as to how the agency and ACT can interface to coordinate and provide consistent services for the client.

14. *Family Member Interview.* Relationship to client of person interviewed; early historical information about the client—anything unusual during gestation or birth; what was the client like as a child—behavior problems, learning problems, relationship with peers; when illness first appeared, etc.; family's knowledge about past treatments and their effect on client; family's relationship with client—frequency of contacts, nature of contacts, help provided to client, help client provides family members, etc.; family's recommendations for the kinds of services they think will be helpful to client; family's willingness to relate to ACT staff regarding client; family's familiarity with the National Alliance for the Mentally Ill and the local chapter.

15. *Interview of Significant Others.* Nature of the relationship; length of the relationship; frequency of contacts; who initiates the contact; assistance to client; client's assistance to significant other; symptoms or unusual behavior noticed when with client; what are the client's strengths and weaknesses; how can ACT be helpful to client; if client is agreeable, willingness to be involved in treatment.

The Comprehensive Treatment Plan

The following paragraphs regarding treatment plan development are adapted from the policy and procedures manual developed by the Gateway ACT team of MHCDC.

The treatment plan will be developed by the primary contact person with input from other team members and other service providers; the client and, if permitted by the client, the family should be involved. Every effort should be made to involve the family in the whole process. If the client initially objects to family involvement, learn why the client objects and help the client and family work it through, so that family involvement is possible. Of course, if these efforts fail and the client still objects to family involvement, the client's wishes must be accepted. However, this may change over time and continued efforts to help the client and family work things through should be made. The client's participation in the development of the plan and goals will be documented in the treatment record or progress note and by the client's signature on the treatment plan. In the event that the client declines to sign his or her plan, a note to that effect will be recorded in the chart by the primary contact person.

The plan will delineate specific goals along with the treatment, rehabilitation, and support service actions necessary to accomplish these goals. The goals shall be developed with both short-term and long-range expectations and shall be written in measurable terms. Inasmuch as possible, the actions shall be client, rather than staff, driven.

Expected outcomes and the staff or agencies responsible for providing the services will be identified on the plan.

Criteria for when any of the specific service actions noted above can be stopped will be described in the plan.

The treatment plan will be included in the clinical record. Treatment and provision of services may begin before the treatment plan is completed.

Once all the preliminary work for the plan is completed and a tentative plan developed, with input from the client, a two-hour meeting is scheduled to finalize the comprehensive plan. Attending this meeting are the team leader, the primary contact person, and the client. If necessary, other staff with special expertise needed by the client should also participate. At this meeting, the final version of the comprehensive treatment plan is developed. It is formally completed when it is reviewed, approved, and signed by the team leader and the psychiatrist.

To give the reader an idea of what a plan might look like, we have created a partial plan utilizing a fictitious client named Mr. John Smith.

Treatment plan for Mr. John Smith:
Primary Contact Person—James Falk

Diagnosis:

Axis I: Schizophrenia Residual Type (295.6); Alcohol Abuse (305.0).
Axis II: None.
Axis III: Allergy to penicillin.
Axis IV: Psychosocial stressors: Recently moved to new apartment; recently had payee appointed to manage money because of increased alcohol use.
Axis V: Current G.A.F.: 50, increased use of alcohol and poor hygiene.
Lowest G.A.F.: 25, brief relapse into psychotic episode.
Highest G.A.F.: 70, symptoms stabilized, not abusing alcohol.

Strengths:

Mr. Smith does accept the fact that he has a mental illness and is willing to take medication. When not abusing alcohol, he is able to shop for food, keep up his apartment, manage his money, and maintain good personal hygiene. Although he is somewhat shy, he relates well with others and is generous by nature. He does enjoy listening to music and has some artistic talent.

Focus Area A: Alcohol Abuse.
Description:

Mr. Smith has a history of periodically using and abusing alcohol. During the past six months, he has been steadily increasing his alcohol intake and has had frequent episodes of intoxication. During some of those episodes he has created a disturbance in his apartment building, leading to eviction. Fortunately, we were able to find a new apartment for him quite quickly. He acknowledges that he is having a problem with alcohol, but feels he needs a lot of help to, as he puts it, "get back on the wagon." During one of his more difficult periods, he stopped taking his medication and began to show the reemergence of psychotic symptoms. We had been monitoring his condition closely and caught it in time to prevent a full-blown episode. To help him get his drinking under control, we found a payee to manage his money, started to give him his medications on a daily basis, and had him reassessed for our alcohol and other drug abuse (AODA) treatment program.

Short-term Goal:

By 9/20/97, he will have completed his AODA assessment, evidenced by case notes.

Short-term Goal:

By 10/20/97, he will be able to manage his medications one week at a time, as evidenced by monitoring his medications and reporting it in the case notes.

Short-term Goal:

By 12/20/97, he will be able to manage money on a weekly basis, with major bills still being paid by his payee, as evidenced both in the case notes and in the money management file.

Long-term Goal:

By 02/01/98, he will be consistently following the recommendations specified in the treatment plan that he and the drug and alcohol abuse specialist developed together, as evidenced by case notes reporting observations made regarding his functioning.

Long-term Goal:

By 2/1/98, he will be able to manage both his money and his medications, as evidenced by the case notes.

Plan:

1. Kate Fried (substance abuse specialist) will continue working with Mr. Smith and keeping the rest of the ACT team informed as to what they might be doing to help facilitate his AODA program. His progress in this area will be discussed every time Mr. Smith's name comes up in the daily meeting when the clients are reviewed.

2. James Falk (primary contact person) will remind Mr. Smith about the money management plan to which he has agreed and stay in close contact with the payee to ensure that the plan is carried out. Mr. Falk will also monitor the situation closely and, if there are problems, Mr. Falk and Mr. Smith will renegotiate the details of the plan.

3. Bill Meld (nurse) will package medication for Mr. Smith to conform to the medication plan noted above. Mr. Falk will monitor closely and renegotiate the plan if necessary.

The example given above is a partial plan that includes just one focus area. However, a full plan would include a focus area for each problem. Thus, it may include problems such as psychiatric symptomatology, activities of daily living, social relationships, vocational, financial, etc. Each problem area would be treated as the example given above for alcohol abuse. That is, each problem area would have a descriptive section, short-term and long-term goal sections with a notation as to how each of the goals will be measured and documented, and finally, specific plans as to who would do what to help bring the goals to fruition. Finally, the treatment plan is signed by the client, the team leader, and the psychiatrist.

Treatment Plan Reviews

The treatment plan must be reviewed and updated every six months for each client and more often when needed. In order to have sufficient treatment planning meetings to accomplish this, the ACT program routinely schedules two two-hour treatment planning meetings per week. On most teams, all team members attend the treatment planning meeting. However, some teams limit attendance at this meeting to the client, the client's primary contact person, and any other person or persons that the primary contact person or the client feels is needed. (This treatment planning meeting is distinct from the daily staff meeting, which is always attended by all staff and will be described later in this chapter). The secretary will notify the primary contact person six weeks prior to the date when the treatment plan update needs to be completed. It is then the primary contact person's responsibility to reserve one of the treatment planning meeting times prior to that date.

By the time of this meeting, it is expected that all the necessary data will have been collected and that a tentative, updated treatment plan will have been developed in concert with the client. This will include the client's progress and current status in meeting the goals set forth in the plan. Goals that have been met will be upgraded, intensified, or deleted, as appropriate.

Goals that have not been met will be lowered to a more realistic level, modified, continued, or deleted, with an explanation given in the case note or review narrative. The treatment plan review shall be recorded in the client's treatment record, including (a) The date and results of the review and any changes in the plan, as well as the explanation for such changes, and (b) The names of participants in the case conference.

The primary contact person then discusses the results of the case review with the client, client's guardian if he or she has one, and with the family if the client consents. Also recorded is the client's or guardian's acknowledgment of any changes in the plan.

Just as with the first comprehensive treatment plan, each treatment plan review must be approved and signed by the team leader and the psychiatrist.

Daily Team Meeting

If the ACT team is the heart of the ACT program, the daily team meeting is its nerve center. It is here that the whole team is kept abreast of what is going on with all the clients. It is here that client problems are discussed, plans made as to what needs to be done, and staff assignments made to carry out the plan. The meeting is held daily, lasts approximately one hour, is held at a time when as many staff as possible can be present. Many ACT teams hold this meeting around the noon hour, when both the morning and evening staff are present (when it is held is less important than ensuring that it is held at a time when all staff can be available). The meeting is chaired by the team leader. The agenda is as follows:

1. Announcements: housekeeping, upcoming community meetings, information from the parent organization that needs to be disseminated to the staff, etc. This section of the meeting is generally short, less than five minutes.

2. A quick review of the nonemergency tasks (e.g., accompanying clients to doctor appointments, getting blood drawn for laboratory analysis, delivering medications, etc.), many of which are routine, that need to be carried out that day and which staff member will be doing them. This section of the meeting is quite short.

3. Addressing urgent client or system issues (on one of the wall boards are the names of clients or issues placed there by any staff member, indicating that these items need the team's attention, that day, at that meeting). As much of the meeting time as needed is taken to deal with these urgent issues. On some days, most of the meeting is occupied with urgent problems; on other days, they may take only a few minutes.

4. General review of clients: In the time remaining (on some days there is very little and on other days there is quite a lot), the roster of clients is reviewed. Beginning with the client at the top, the roster is reviewed until the meeting time is over. Note is taken where in the roster the meeting ended, so that the next day, when this section of the meeting commences, the next client in line is reviewed. Using this system, every client is briefly reviewed about twice a week. This is an absolutely crucial exercise because it ensures that no one is neglected. If, for example, a name is read and the staff does not know how that client is doing across all the important variables (housing, finances, health, socialization, etc.), an assignment will be made to find the client and review all these areas so that the team will know what it must do, if anything, to help that client achieve the goal of a stable life of decent quality in the community.

Monitoring clients is absolutely essential for an ACT program; without it staff action is haphazard. The daily meeting ensures that this monitoring function is being done and that all staff are kept abreast of every client. When the meeting ends, the staff go out to carry out their assignments and the secretary remains behind to respond to calls, take messages, and do routine work. If a situation arises that requires a professional staff member's response, the secretary uses the paging system to contact the appropriate staff person. On those teams where not everyone carries a pager, the secretary, who routinely attends the daily meeting, has some information as to where the various staff are and tries to locate them.

Many of the staff assignments are routine: delivering medications to a client who takes them on a daily basis but is unwilling to come to the ACT office to pick them up; going to a client's apartment to help him or her learn the activities necessary to live independently; going to the hospital to assess and work with a client and collaborate with the inpatient team on treatment and discharge planning; taking a client to his doctor's appointment for a medical problem and helping the client understand and follow through with the doctor's recommendation; taking a client to the Social Security office and helping the client apply for benefits; etc. Below are three examples of how ACT staff deal with some problems that are not quite routine but not infrequent. These examples come from the authors' experience working with successful ACT programs and are provided here to give the reader some idea of the mind-set an ACT program must adopt when working with clients in the community.

Keeping Clients from Dropping Out of the Program

Keeping clients involved with the program is of paramount importance. Frequently, patients with severe and persistent mental illness do not seem to be motivated to stay involved with treatment. What is often most frustrating about their willingness to be involved is that it is highly variable. There are times when a client will seek help; at other times, the same client does not want to have anything to do with the treatment program. When treatment personnel, being fired by a client, accept this with a shrug of their shoulders and a comment that "unmotivated people can't be helped," they show poor clinical judgment. Lack of or variability in motivation is part of the basic illness. If this lack is accepted passively, there is a high probability that the client will again face psychosis in a relatively short period of time, be hospitalized, and be referred back at discharge to start all over again.

ACT programs must be assertive in keeping clients involved. If someone does not show up for an appointment or for a job, it will be highlighted to be discussed at the daily meeting. The person who has a good relationship with the client at that moment in time (it might or might not be the primary contact person) is given the assignment of going out and finding the client. The staff person may have to go to his home or drive along the street where the client frequents. When he is found, he is invited to go for a cup of coffee (the staff person will be willing to pay for it) where the staff person tries to learn why he missed the appointment and to find out from the client how the ACT program can help him make his appointments in the future. The client may insist that he wants no help and that the ACT team should just leave him alone. The staff then acknowledges that the client appears angry with the team and then tries to find out what was is bothering him. This must be done in a nondefensive manner. The staff person may say that the ACT team really wants to be helpful and that, if the team offended the client in some way, the team would like to know what happened and to explain or, if the situation warrants it, apologize. The staff person stresses that the team wants to be of continued help. The main message, given over and over, is that the team really does care about what happens to the client and is there to help the client. The client may respond by saying he doesn't want any help from the team. The staff person responds by saying he understands that is how the client is feeling today, but he will be back tomorrow to check in with the client. The experience of ACT programs in situations like this is that with persistent effort the client will eventually come back into the program. In addition, over time, clients do learn that, perhaps unlike past experiences, this team will go out of its way to be helpful and so must really care. This approach has very significantly reduced dropouts from ACT programs.

Focusing on Clients' Strengths

We have learned that clients do much better if we, in addition to treating their pathology, pay a good deal of attention to their strengths.

Mr. Jones was a 35-year-old single man with a fixed paranoid delusional system. A variety of psychotropic medications at different dosage levels had been tried, but he remained delusional. However, his delusion was quite circumscribed, and his reality testing for activities of daily living was good. Even when actively delusional, he had no history of being either verbally or physically threatening or violent.

Mr. Jones had a good work history prior to developing his paranoid psychosis. He was a skilled auto mechanic and, because of his energetic nature, his production level was high and of good quality. However, since becoming symptomatic he had been unable to keep a job. At times he would get agitated when his delusional thinking became more than he could tolerate and he would begin talking loudly to himself. This was not tolerated well by employers or fellow employees and he would be fired.

The treatment staff concluded that to help Mr. Jones keep his job, they would need to give a good deal of support to his employer and actively teach the employer to pay attention to Mr. Jones's productivity rather than just his talking loudly to himself. After a search, they found an employer who was willing to give him a try. With Mr. Jones's permission, they gave the employer some information about his psychiatric problem and assured him that Mr. Jones was not dangerous. The staff also assured the employer that they would be available to help any time he felt he needed their assistance. Further, they suggested that he focus primarily on Mr. Jones's work effort and try to ignore his habit of talking to himself.

During Mr. Jones's first week of work, the employer called the staff several times when Mr. Jones started talking to himself more loudly than usual. Each time, the staff came immediately, assessed Mr. Jones, and reassured the employer that the situation was in hand. As the weeks progressed, Mr. Jones became less anxious in his work and the employer became less anxious about him. The calls from the employer decreased significantly. Months later, Mr. Jones continued to work and the staff continued to respond to the employer's rare requests for an immediate assessment of the client. In this case, focusing on the client's strengths rather than just on his pathology brought large dividends in a rehabilitation effort.

Relating to Clients as Responsible Citizens

In order to work effectively with clients as well as with the community, the staff must embrace the attitude that the people they are working with are first and foremost citizens of the community, that they are living in the community because it is their right and not because the community is allowing them to be there, that patients are, indeed, free agents able to make decisions and be responsible for their actions. These attitudes influence clinical behaviors.

One area where this is important involves medications. Clients are frequently ambivalent about taking medications. We find we get better compliance if we relate to clients as responsible persons. As much as possible, we collaborate with them regarding medication decisions. While we certainly try to influence clients' decisions, we do not fight with them or attempt to control them regarding medication decisions when we do not have the power to do so. We are willing to negotiate about dosage and to set a range within which clients can control their own dosages according to their needs. At times, we agree to clients' requests for small changes in medications that we believe are pharmacologically insignificant (though some clients do respond markedly to very small dose changes) because we know this gives clients a real and important sense of control and participation in their treatment. Further, we respect clients' knowledge of what is going on in their bodies. This approach makes them a part of the treatment process and shows respect for them as responsible persons.

Another important clinical reason to treat clients as responsible citizens is that some have learned that they can use their illness as an excuse for their behavior. We disabuse our clients of that notion. We tell them that we believe that they are ill (otherwise we would not be prescribing medication or providing other treatment), but that we do not believe they should use their illness as an excuse for unacceptable behavior. We tell them that we will do everything we can to see to it that their positive behaviors are rewarded, but that for their negative behaviors they should get the same consequences that we would receive had we behaved that way.

As an example, we had one client who believed he should be rehospitalized whenever he became even mildly stressed or anxious. His way of accomplishing that would be to go into a supermarket, take some soda and candy, and walk through the line without paying for it. If he were not apprehended, he would simply walk back in and take more until someone called the police. He would then get into the police car and half a block down the road would say to the policeman, "Oh, by the way, I'm a patient at the state hospital." At this point, the policeman would sigh with relief, turn the car around, and give him a free taxi ride to the hospital. The policeman not only thought he was doing a good thing but also avoided having to take him downtown, book him, write a detailed report, show up in court, and so on. To avoid the problem of the police taxiing the client to the hospital, we had to work very closely not only with the police but also with the district attorney and the judges to see to it that this kind of minor crime was handled as it would be for any other citizen. The next time this client shoplifted at a supermarket he went before a judge; the judge gave him the same stern lecture he gives to all first offenders of this crime. The judge told him, "If you ever do this again you will spend three days in the county jail or have a $50.00 fine." For most people (and most clients) this would be sufficient to stop the behavior. However, this client shoplifted again, and since he didn't have $50.00, he spent three days in the county jail. Our staff spent a good deal of those three days in the jail as well, working not only with the client but also with the jailers to make sure everyone got through the three days all right. With this approach, we found that the client's maladaptive style of coping with stress dropped precipitously.

We do not advocate this approach for people who break the law in the midst of a psychotic episode. We must use good clinical judgment to determine when this approach should be used. Because we do this with clients whom we know well, we have little difficulty in determining when our clients are consciously breaking the law as a maladaptive coping strategy and when they are doing things because they are really out of touch with reality.

Money Management

At times, it is absolutely essential that the team help the client manage his money. Many clients have not learned the coping skills required to develop and keep to a budget. When this is the case, most clients will voluntarily cooperate with the ACT team in a money management program. As the client learns budgeting skills, the amount of money he or she manages over a specific time period is increased, in a gradual fashion, until he/she is able to handle all of it independently. The other extreme is a drug dependent client who uses the major portion of his or her money to buy drugs and neglects mandatory expenditures such as rent and food. In cases like this it is often necessary to legally get a payee to cooperate with the ACT team in the management of the client's money. Some teams act as payee while other teams have someone outside the team act as payee. In any case, the arrangement necessitates that the payee, no matter who it is, cooperate with the team in money management. In extreme cases, the client gets no cash at all. His major bills—rent, phone, etc.—are paid, and the client gets vouchers for items such as food and cigarettes. In order to accomplish this, the team must develop relationships with local merchants who will sell the vouchers to the team and only give the client the products for which the vouchers have been purchased. There are a number of situations, between the two extremes given above, where helping the client manage money is extremely useful. Needless to say, a careful accounting system must be maintained to ensure that the client gets all the money entitled to him or her. In addition, an audit by the parent agency should be conducted periodically to ensure that this activity is being handled in a very scrupulous manner.

Discharge Criteria

It is useful to have an established discharge process and a system to arrange for necessary follow-up or follow-along care for clients who meet discharge criteria. This is consistent with the principle that the ACT team serves as the fixed point of responsibility for the clients in its program. Thus, when someone is discharged, it is the responsibility of the ACT team to ensure that the service the client will be using can appropriately serve his or her needs. Further, the ACT team continues to monitor and provide services when necessary, until the client is firmly involved with the new service. It is not until this transitioning process is successfully completed that the ACT team relinquishes its role as the fixed point of responsibility for the client.

The following are the procedures utilized by the Gateway ACT team of the Mental Health Center of Dane County, Inc.:

1. Each client will have established, agreed-upon discharge criteria that are understood to signify the progress the client is to have made before discharge from the program would ordinarily be considered.

2. Discharge criteria will be reviewed at each treatment plan review period and as needed.

3. An individual can be discharged from the program for the following reasons:

   a. death;

   b. a move out of the geographic area of responsibility;

   c. a move into a nursing home, permanently, for medical reasons;

   d. sentenced with a prison term of long duration;

   e. able to function well with less intensive or comprehensive services and acceptance of care responsibilities by another provider capable of meeting the client's current needs. Plus, a plan for transition and follow-up to ensure that the client has established a firm connection with the new program and that the services are, indeed, adequate.

4. When the client approaches completion of discharge criteria goals, the primary contact person will begin discussions with the client about the process of discharge and what discharge plan needs to be put in place.

5. Referrals to other services will be made, if needed, and those services will accept the person into their programs before the ACT program's discharge is completed. In the rare event that other services are not necessary, a plan for follow-up to assess how the person is doing without ACT services will be established.

6. Documentation by the client's primary contact person, team leader, and psychiatrist of the client's discharge from ACT will be entered in the client's treatment record upon termination of treatment services. Documentation of discharge will include:

   a. the reasons for discharge;

   b. the client's status and condition at discharge;

   c. a written final evaluation summary of the client's progress toward the goals set forth in the treatment plan;

   d. a plan developed, in conjunction with the client, for care after discharge and for follow-up;

   e. the signature of the primary contact person, team leader, and psychiatrist.

Not mentioned among the discharge criteria is the simple wish of the client to be discharged from the service. It is not unusual for clients in ACT programs to express a wish to be discharged. The fact of the matter is that this is very rarely a simple matter. Clients chosen for ACT programs are generally the most difficult to treat in the system and it has been demonstrated numerous times that other programs have not been successful in helping them stabilize and improve their lives. The ACT program is not easy for clients; it is a demanding program, but the program always provides staff to support and help the client manage the demands. Nevertheless, clients at times feel overwhelmed and, in the moment, demand to be discharged. Earlier in this chapter, an example was given of how to respond to this kind of problem. There are times, however, albeit rare, that this approach does not work and the client continues to insist that he or she wants nothing further to do with the program. This situation almost never occurs with a client who will do well without the program; if that were the case, the normal discharge procedure described above would be put into effect. The client demanding discharge will almost surely deteriorate and relapse into psychosis without the involvement of the ACT program. What should the ACT team do in this case? We recommend the following:

a. Do not discharge the client.

b. Continue periodic contacts with the client in an attempt to persuade him or her to return to the program.

c. Stay in close touch with the client's family and others who are close to the client, both to get information on how the client is doing and to provide support to them during this very stressful time.

d. Continue to help the client in any way possible, through collaterals, if not directly.

e. When the client's condition deteriorates to the point of requiring involuntary treatment, help the appropriate parties institute the legal procedures necessary to get the client back into treatment.

f. If the client is involuntarily hospitalized, go to the hospital and work with the inpatient staff, as well as with the client; have the hospitalization be as short as possible and continue working with the client after discharge.

g. Help the client, in the most supportive way possible, learn from this experience and try and get the client to recommend what should be done if it happens again.

Ensuring Model Adherence

Research has shown a strong correlation between ACT program effectiveness and fidelity to the ACT model. The Dartmouth ACT Fidelity Scale, an unpublished instrument developed at the New Hampshire Dartmouth Psychiatric Research Center, Lebanon, New Hampshire, in 1995 by Teague, Drake, and Bond, provides a means of measuring fidelity to the ACT model. This scale looks at the ACT model utilizing three domains: the structure and composition of human resources, the organizational boundaries of the program, and the nature of the services it provides. The following paragraphs give some of the dimensions of these domains. The dimensions given represent the highest degree of fidelity. Most ACT programs do not reach this degree of fidelity in all areas, but to be effective the ACT program must come close to many of them.

Human Resources: Structure and Composition

1. The caseload should be small, optimally, with a client-to-staff ratio no greater than ten-to-one.

2. The staff operate as a team, rather than as individual practitioners, and all the staff know and work with all the clients.

3. There are frequent team meetings to plan and review services for each client. Optimally, the team reviews each client daily, even if only briefly.

4. The team leader is also involved in direct service, optimally, at least 50 percent of the time.

5. The turnover of staff is low so that there is high continuity of staffing for clients, optimally less than 20 percent turnover in two years.

6. Once the team is fully operational, it is rare for the team to not be fully staffed. Optimally, the team has operated at 95 percent capacity in the past 12 months.

7. A psychiatrist is assigned to the team with adequate time to follow the clients, plus sufficient time to participate in some staff meetings; optimally, there is a half-time psychiatrist for every fifty clients.

8. There are sufficient nurses, substance abuse specialists, and vocational specialists on the team to meet clients' needs in those areas, optimally a full-time staff person in each of the above positions for every fifty clients.

Organizational Boundaries

1. There are explicit admission criteria and the team has, and uses, measurable and operationally defined criteria to screen out inappropriate referrals.

2. The intake rate is low enough to maintain a stable service environment, optimally no more than six admissions per month.

3. Optimally, the team provides a full array of services, including psychiatric, alcohol and other drug abuse treatment, vocational rehabilitation, housing support, counseling/psychotherapy, and a host of other supportive and practical help services required by the client to make a stable life in the community.

4. The team has twenty-four-hour responsibility for covering crises.

5. The team is responsible for hospital admissions, working with the inpatient team in treatment and discharge planning.

6. The team provides time-unlimited services by remaining the point of contact for all clients, as needed.

Nature of Services

1. The team spends most of its time, optimally 80 percent, working in the community, monitoring client status and helping clients develop community living skills in vivo rather than in the office.

2. The ACT program has a no dropout policy; 95 percent or more of the case load is retained in a twelve-month period.

3. The team is assertive in keeping clients engaged in the program and consistently demonstrates well-thought-out strategies, including legal mechanisms when appropriate, to keep clients engaged with the program.

4. The ACT team provides intensive services, in terms of time spent with clients, optimally an average of two hours per week or more per client.

5. There is a high frequency of contact with clients, optimally an average of four or more contacts per week per client.

6. The ACT team provides supports for client's support network—family, friends, landlords, employers, etc.—optimally one contact per week or more per client, with support system in the community.

7. The ACT program uses a stage-wise treatment model that is nonconfrontational, follows behavioral principles, considers interactions of mental illness and substance abuse, and has gradual expectations of abstinence. Optimally, clients with substance abuse disorders spend twenty-four minutes or more per week in substance abuse treatment; at least 50 percent of the clients with substance abuse attend at least one substance abuse treatment group meeting during the month and the above treatments are provided by ACT staff.

Guidelines for Starting a New ACT Team

When an organization makes the decision to develop an ACT program there are a number of useful guidelines. First, the organization must clearly have in mind what role it wants the ACT program to play in the overall treatment system. This will facilitate the development of specific client admission criteria for the program. Second, the parent organization should educate the other service providers in the organization and other potential referral sources outside of the organization about the ACT program. Included in that education is a description of appropriate client referrals, what the goal of the program will be for those clients, and, very importantly, that ACT operates with a service integration model and thus most of the services needed by those clients will be provided by the ACT team. It should be made explicitly clear that referrals to the ACT team will necessitate the transition of clients from the psychiatrists and therapists of the referral source to the ACT team.

In hiring the ACT staff it is a good idea to hire the team leader first and have the team leader fully involved in all future hirings. The team leader must be a well trained mental health professional who has considerable knowledge about working with persons who have a serious and persistent mental illness. Optimally, the team leader would be someone who has worked on an ACT team. If that is not possible, then it must be someone who has several years of experience working with severely mentally ill people in the community. In addition to the professional training and experience, the team leader must have the personal qualities to inspire his or her team members to do the kind of difficult, but very professionally rewarding, work ACT requires. These qualities are described in detail in the Chapter 7.

The next hires should be a part-time psychiatrist, nurse, and clinician (we recommend a masters level psychiatric social worker). It is not too important in what order those three are hired; what is important is that they, like the team leader, be professionally competent and have the personal characteristics that would make them team players. As these professionals come on board, they should be involved in future hirings. The next step is to find a well functioning ACT program that is willing to have the four staff visit to see firsthand how an ACT team operates and possibly to establish a consultative relationship with the team leader.

The parent organization must now make available the physical needs of the team—adequate space, telephones, office furniture, office equipment, etc. By this time, the team has developed the forms and record system it will be using, borrowing from the team they visited and/or using the forms in the appendix of this book. In all likelihood, the parent organization has clinical forms that are routinely used for their purposes, some of which will have to be employed by the team.

The team is now ready to begin accepting clients. The clients must be *taken in at a slow rate,* primarily for two reasons: One, the clients themselves require a great deal of time since they are persons with high needs and are often relatively unstable; and two, as is clear from the material earlier in this chapter, the assessment and treatment planning activities are very time-consuming. It is recommended that the rate not exceed five, at most six, per month. In addition, as the caseload increases, there may be times when the rate of intake has to be temporarily decreased below five per month.

As the caseload increases, there must be a commensurate increase in the size of the staff. The order of the remainder of the hirings will be dependent on the needs of the already admitted clients, as well as the availability of the needed staff. These include a drug and alcohol treatment specialist, vocational specialist, and secretary. As we made clear in describing the staff, we cannot overemphasize the value of a good secretary. Thus, do not wait too long before filling that position. The total number of staff hired will be determined by how many clients the program is planning to have and the client-to-staff ratio the program decides to use. This ratio should not exceed ten-to-one (keep in mind that the secretary and psychiatrist are not counted in this ratio). We recommend that the total number of clients not exceed one hundred.

As the staff size increases, it is advisable for the staff who have not visited the consulting ACT team to do so. It is also important to receive continued consultation from that team and from other experts in operating ACT programs. Getting specialized consultation from experts in subprograms within ACT, such as drug and alcohol abuse treatment and vocational rehabilitation, is very useful. The new program can be considered a mature program after it has attained a full complement of clients and staff and has been operating with them for at least two years. This program is now in a position to provide consultation to emerging ACT programs. However, mature programs should also have consultation available to them from other mature programs; the need for consultation never ends.

Suggested Readings

Diamond, R. J. (1983). Enhancing medication use in schizophrenic patients. *Journal of Clinical Psychiatry, 44*(2), 7.

Stein, L. I., & Diamond, R. J. (1985). The chronic mentally ill and the criminal justice system: When to call the police. *Hospital & Community Psychiatry, 36*, 271–274.

Stein, L. I., & Test, M. A., (1985). Training in community living model: A decade of experience. *New Directions for Mental Health Services, 26.*

▸▸▸❯ 10 ❰◂◂◂◂

Rural, Dually Diagnosed, and Homeless Populations

This chapter addresses four timely and policy-relevant issues associated with the dissemination of ACT services. Specifically discussed are key modifications and adaptations necessary to implement effective ACT programs (1) in rural settings, (2) for homeless populations, (3) to maximize employment opportunities, and (4) to minimize the use of illicit drugs.

Vocational Rehabilitation

The importance of work in a person's life cannot be overemphasized. Work is the most important determinant of a person's identity and self-confidence. It provides a way to structure one's time and gives a sense of daily purpose. It facilitates social relationships, social support, and the building of networks in the course of one's life. In the process of rehabilitation and recovery, nothing can substitute for work in terms of its impact on a person's sense of well-being.

While most individuals with severe mental disorders are interested in work as an important goal for themselves, mental health professionals tend to discourage this ambition. For the vast majority of mental health providers and administrators, the assumption of unemployment goes hand-in-hand with their beliefs about the course of severe mental illness and its poor potential for rehabilitation. As a rule, the majority of both private and public "state of the art" mental health systems and programs do not consider work a directly targeted outcome of their efforts. Further, clients who receive social insurance benefits for their mental disability are understandably reluctant to give up their eligibility for what may be low-paying jobs with little chance for advancement. Consequently, the unemployment rate among persons with severe mental illness has remained around 85 percent, double that of those with severe physical disabilities.

Criteria commonly used to evaluate the success of mental health treatment and rehabilitation programs generally do not include work. If a mental health system or program endorses the importance of work in a person's rehabilitation process, it must have the capacity to assist clients to achieve functional outcomes that include work. Such outcomes range from work in the family setting to community volunteerism to competitive employment. Work as an outcome is arguably the single most important marker of the success of any treatment/rehabilitation system or program that markets itself as "state of the art" in facilitating the community integration of persons with severe and persistent mental illness.

There are other major barriers to vocational rehabilitation. The federal and state vocational rehabilitation programs, created by Congress in 1920 and revised in 1943 to specifically address the needs of severely mentally ill populations, have failed miserably in achieving their intended aims with regard to this population. Resources available from federal and state vocational rehabilitation funds are directed toward client assessment and/or administrative activities such as eligibility determination. In these vast bureaucracies there appears to be little interest in using financial resources to directly assist severely mentally ill clients in acquiring and keeping jobs. The agency's usual orientation is toward time-limited assistance and, as such, is contrary to what is known about the need to provide time-unlimited services for this population. The agency rewards its vocational counselors for focusing efforts on individuals with much less severe mental disorders, who are not likely to require much on-the-job assistance. In addition, vocational counselors are poorly trained about recent developments in our understanding of the biological nature of severe mental illness. We know that severe mental illnesses have a biological basis, that is, that there is an abnormality in the central nervous system responsible for the etiology and maintenance of the disorder. This underlying pathology leads to impairment in, loss or reduction of certain functions, such as a person's capacity to remain task-oriented and to discriminate social cues, skills that nonmentally ill people take for granted and that are crucial to gaining and maintaining competitive employment.

The History of Vocational Rehabilitation Programs

In the United States, a variety of program approaches have been used in an effort to provide vocational rehabilitation and/or daytime structure to the lives of persons with severe mental illnesses (see Table 10-1). Only in recent years, however, has the possibility of real employment been seriously considered by policymakers as a desirable and achievable outcome of services to persons with severe mental illnesses.

The history of post-institutionalization vocational rehabilitation efforts and "model" approaches in the United States has been succinctly summarized by Bond (1992). He categorized progress in the development of various approaches into three general "eras":

1. *1950s–1960s: The Rule of Imperial Institutions.* During this period, "vocational programs were implemented in hospitals, sheltered workshops, and halfway houses . . . the optimism that prompted these facility-based efforts was soon overtaken by a deeply felt pessimism about the employment potential for psychiatric patients. . . ." Remnants of this era remain prevalent today in the form of "day hospitals," "day care programs," "partial hospital programs," and "rehabilitative day treatment programs." These approaches provide an efficient mechanism for a variety of staff to deliver a range of mostly medical and recreational services in a central location and in a lucrative manner, as these are usually billable services for most insurance providers. This is a popular service approach, in that the range of usual hospital services can continue to be provided by the hospital multidisciplinary team at a lower cost than full hospital-based (overnight) programs. Their serious drawback is that they keep clients in a segregated environment and, as such, fail to directly assist in facilitating community integration by directly promoting the development of community natural support networks, social integration, and daytime activities in natural, community environments.

2. *1970s–1980s: The Dark Ages.* During this period, Bond writes, "vocational rehabilitation for persons with severe mental illness was not considered the mission of either community mental health centers or comprehensive vocational rehabilitation centers. Psychosocial rehabilitation centers such as Fountain House (New York, New York), Horizon House (Philadelphia, Pennsylvania), and The Club (Piscataway, New Jersey) developed transitional employment programs. These programs were seen either as 'maverick' or as 'model', depending on one's ideology. They existed as isolated fiefdoms within nonvocational-oriented mental health systems. . . ." These programs are less symptom-oriented in their treatment approaches than partial hospital programs and provide greater emphasis on socialization and the learning of new psychosocial skills. Their design, however, falls short of potentially achieving full community integration for their clients, since skills learned in these settings may not generalize to a person's natural community environment. In addition, employment is time-limited and program staff do not provide continued support and assistance in the com-

munity beyond transitional employment. As such, this approach is inconsistent with "gold-standard" rehabilitation program outcomes, which call for full community integration in real-life settings.

3. *1990s–present: A Renaissance.* The beginning of the present period was marked by mental health providers using an approach borrowed from the field of mental retardation. This approach, known as "supported employment," moved the service site from facility-based to field-based settings. This reflected a true paradigm shift; it was a movement away from an emphasis on prevocational training to directly placing people in real jobs and supporting them on the job. Preliminary research on this approach has led to a heightened sense of hope about our rehabilitation efforts. The main point of current debate between "old guard" providers and "renaissance" providers in the field of vocational rehabilitation is one of service-site specificity:

a. Whether to provide vocational rehabilitation services within facilities operated by hospitals, rehabilitation agencies, or through business subcontract enclaves where all co-workers are persons with mental illnesses; or
b. To provide assistance in "real-world" competitive work sites in settings where the mentally disabled persons are integrated with nondisabled workers, in positions that are open to anyone and pay wages comparable to those paid to other employees in the same position.

As highlighted in Table 10-1, in the absence of present-day consensus, the field is replete with service programs in both categories. The entire range of programs listed in Table 10-1 can be found across the nation today. The specific type of program found in a given community is influenced by state and local policy and the views of mental health administrators and professionals on whether vocational services should be facility-based or field-based.

Table 10-1
Vocational Rehabilitation Models for Persons with Severe Mental Illness

Facility-Based Models	Field-Based (Supported Employment) Models
Vocational Counseling	Assertive Community Treatment
Hospital-based Inpatient Programs	Individual Placement and Support
Partial Hospital Programs	Case Management *plus* Supported Employment
Sheltered Workshops	Transitional Employment *plus* Supported Employment
Halfway Houses (Fairweather Lodges)	Psychosocial Rehabilitation *plus* Supported Employment
Enclaves (subcontract work crews)	
Job Clubs	
Psychosocial Rehabilitation Centers	

Research on these vocational rehabilitation approaches suggests that the facility-based programs in the first column of Table 10-1 often place people in jobs for which they are poorly prepared and rarely provide continued support at a real work site beyond the walls of their program. As such, facility-based programs that do not provide assistance in real work sites can claim only modest success in employing persons with severe mental illnesses. Further, they may be unwittingly setting up clients for possible failure and humiliation. On the other hand, research on field-based programs that provide continued and comprehensive employment assistance and support at a real work site (second column of Table 10-1) suggests that this approach yields a greater chance of maintaining job success. This is especially true in obtaining competitive employment positions. This concept of providing long-term support and assistance continuously at a work site is known as "supported employment." This is a "place-then-train" approach to job attainment and retention, in contrast to the "train-then-place" sequence used in traditional vocational and psychosocial rehabilitation programs.

You will note in Table 10-1 that field-based approaches include those that combine traditional models, such as case management and psychosocial rehabilitation programs, with supported employment initiatives. This trend toward practical solutions rather than ideology is encouraging.

The supported employment movement is gaining acceptance. This is in part due to the public's increasing hunger for evidence-based approaches and related frustration with the mental health field's tendency to hang on to untested theories of human behavior and psychosocial treatments. These theories are often promulgated in professional training programs with little change over time.

The potential for improved employment outcomes through supported employment has prompted a trend toward community mental health agencies taking responsibility for vocational rehabilitation services. In some states, certification standards require treatment teams to include vocational specialists. These initiatives have been greatly facilitated through the work of the National Alliance for the Mentally Ill, whose efforts are gradually increasing the general public's support for the full community integration of persons with severe mental illnesses. The recent passage of the Americans with Disabilities Act has begun to further community integration by gradually facilitating employer collaboration at a national level.

Research also provides indications about other general predictors of success and failure. Predictors of success include prior work experience, prior work pride, expectation to work, lower rates of hospitalizations in recent years, higher levels of functioning, residential stability, low community unemployment rates, and continued assistance and support at the work site. Predictors of failure include poor interviewing skills, clinical diagnosis of schizophrenia, recipients of SSI/SSDI, and high community unemployment rates. Success is associated with community unemployment rates of less than 2 percent, while failure is associated with rates above 6 percent. These predictors may be useful in improving planning for services to optimize outcomes. As an example, in order to maximize community integration of the largest number of mentally ill persons in an area with low-to-medium unemployment rates, a service system might target clients with prior employment histories who meet other known predictive criteria for living successfully in communities. On the other hand, for clients known to meet predictor criteria for failure, facility-based programs would be made available, initially, in an effort to structure their day as a prevocational initiative.

Vocational Approaches and Assertive Community Treatment

Vocational rehabilitation in ACT is a continuous process; that is, each work experience adds knowledge about the client's interest and abilities. The vocational specialist thus helps the client to integrate these experiences and use them to make the next step more successful.

The vocational rehabilitation approach used most often in the context of ACT is known as "supported employment." In supported employment, ACT staff work with clients at the actual employment site. They provide as much and whatever type of support and assistance the client needs in order to obtain and keep a job or to move on to another one. They provide support and encouragement, job and social skills training, close monitoring of job performance, and mediate difficulties with co-workers and employers serving as the client's advocate. There are two popular "models" for providing supported employment services for ACT clients. These two models differ primarily in the degree to which vocational specialists are integrated into the rest of the work of the ACT team and whether or not the vocational specialists are involved in nonvocational activities with clients:

Model 1. The Program of Assertive Community Treatment (PACT) Integrated Vocational Rehabilitation Approach (PACT IVR). This approach was developed at the Mendota Mental Health Institute in Madison, Wisconsin, and has been the practice at the Program of Assertive Community Treatment in Madison since 1985. This is a total team approach in which all ACT clinical staff share responsibility for providing employment services. The

vocational specialists on the team also share responsibility for clinical and case management activities. There is emphasis by the whole team on vocational rehabilitation as a critical treatment modality and work is viewed as a key need for most clients. The employment specialists have more highly developed interest and knowledge in vocational rehabilitation and job development, which other team members draw upon. However, vocational outcome is a team responsibility, rather than the domain of subspecialists on the team. The vocational specialists on ACT teams have expertise in job development, job placement, job coaching, and providing job support, which includes working with the clients' employers and fellow employees. The vocational specialists on the team must be well suited to developing community employment opportunities.

Model 2. The Individual Placement and Support (IPS) Approach. This approach was designed to be used for a larger population of clients rather than exclusively for ACT team clients. Typically, IPS is established as a specific program within a larger community support system. Staff is headed by a vocational coordinator who has administrative responsibility for the IPS program, serves as primary liaison between it and other programs and services, and supervises several other employment specialists (one for every twenty-five clients). Although the employment specialists are each responsible for a specific caseload, they work as a team to insure uninterrupted vocational services during vacations or staff turnover. Clients assigned to IPS retain their mental health providers and other program assignments. The employment specialist, while focused on employment-related support, must take the initiative to ensure that other clinical staff working with IPS vocational clients support and facilitate the agreed-upon objectives of the client and the IPS worker. IPS was developed specifically to adapt the PACT IVR approach to the environment of most community mental health centers. IPS has been implemented in connection with research projects in New Hampshire and Washington, DC.

Both approaches described above stress direct attainment of competitive employment as the preferred pathway to mastering job skills. Trial employment and volunteer activities in natural community settings are used only if competitive employment options are limited or impossible due to an individual's mental condition. Both use assertive outreach by staff to keep clients involved in treatment and vocational endeavors. Both provide ongoing employment support in the context of a long-term service perspective. They differ with respect to how the employment interventions are integrated, or bundled, with other community support services. That is, they differ in the locus of accountability for vocational outcome and role differentiation among the vocational, treatment, and case management personnel from whom each client receives services (see Table 10-2). These approaches are currently being used in controlled services research settings. They both appear to be significantly more effective than traditional models of vocational rehabilitation.

Table 10-2
Differences Between the IPS and PACT-IVR Supported Employment (S.E.) Models

Service Dimension	PACT- IVR	IPS
Locus of responsibility for S.E. services (job development, job support, etc.).	All ACT staff advised by vocational specialists who are full-time ACT team members.	Separate vocational specialists who are not full-time ACT staff.
Is responsibility for S.E. services shared among vocational specialists and ACT staff?	Yes, vocational specialists are ACT team members.	No, vocational specialists hold all the responsibility.
Usual frequency of contact between vocational specialists and ACT staff.	Daily	Variable
Who receives ACT services?	All ACT clients	Subgroup selected
Do the vocational specialists provide clinical case management services to ACT clients?	Yes	No
Do the clinical case managers provide S.E. services to ACT clients?	Yes	No
Duration of S.E. services	Ongoing	Ongoing
Vocational service site	Field	Field

In summary, we know that, when clients are employed, it is very important to provide them with continuous support, closely monitor for illness relapse, and be ready to provide field-based crisis intervention. We know that in certain work settings clients are likely to become anxious, tense, and overwhelmed; in such situations they may unnecessarily provoke predicaments with co-workers or supervisors. It is imperative, therefore, for co-workers, supervisors, and employers to be knowledgeable about clients' impairments resulting from their mental disorder. In addition, they must feel assured that the employee will receive ongoing assistance from the program and that program staff will respond immediately to a crisis situation. In all the current supported employment models, it is up to the rehabilitation professionals to contact employers and gain their collaboration; this is greatly facilitated by providing convincing evidence that they will remain highly accessible for on-site support.

Rural ACT

The rehabilitation options recently made available under Medicaid have considerably broadened community care and treatment and permitted some states to implement rural outreach as a matter of policy. For example, the State Mental Health Authority of Wisconsin supported the flexible, widespread dissemination of ACT throughout rural Wisconsin. State mental health authorities of Oregon and Michigan have implemented similar rural programs based on ACT principles. Rural outreach is now more timely than ever. Both state mental health authorities and private insurers are seriously attempting to reduce costs associated with hospital use. This trend will encourage both urban and rural approaches to preventing costly hospitalizations.

Among the obstacles associated with implementing rural ACT services are difficulties regarding staff recruitment and retention. The nature of rural outreach requires staff who are naturally inclined to this type of work. The demands of the job, including extensive travel and the absence of the in-office camaraderie more common in traditional settings, make staff recruitment and retention difficult. On the other hand, we have found that certain mental health professionals seem especially well-suited for rural work. A background in home health care, a love of the outdoors, and a distaste for the limits of office-bound work contribute to a good worker-setting match. Clearly, hiring high quality staff is the most critical variable in implementing a successful program. However, if rural jobs are not accompanied by significant incentives, recruiting staff will be difficult.

Differences between Urban and Rural ACT Programs

How ACT operates in rural, compared to urban, areas depends on differences with regard to staff mobility, accessibility, communications, health expectations, attitudes toward treatment, means of transportation, and community resources (see Table 10-3).

As an example, pay telephones, automobile service stations, and other resources that one takes for granted in urban settings are not readily available in rural areas. Cellular phones, important tools of urban teams, may not work reliably in remote areas.

The daily rural-service route requires thoughtful planning. At first, staff may need to travel in teams of two and leave behind a detailed itinerary at a central office. In locations where staff are very familiar with patients and their families and neighbors, one team member may be dropped off at a client's home while the partner visits a nearby site.

TABLE 10-3
Differences between Traditional Services, Urban ACT, and Rural ACT

Service Element	Traditional Services	Urban ACT	Rural ACT
Provider	individual clinician	team	team and community volunteers
Caseload Shared	no	yes	yes
Caseload size	1:50	1:10	1:10
Team rounds	N/A	Daily	Twice weekly
Staff Availability	workday hours	24 hours/7 days	Daytime only[a]
Site	clinics	field	field
Contact Frequency	every 1-3 months	1-3 days	once a week[b]
Family Involvement	occasional	frequent	coincides with home visit
Medication Monitoring	by family	by staff	by staff, family, neighbors, etc.
Housing Arrangements	by client and family	by staff	by staff, family, neighbors, etc.
Case Management Function	broker of services	provider of services	broker and provider
Resource Mobilization	+ effort	++ effort	+++ effort

[a] 24-hour-a-day telephone access—team is responsible for arranging emergency protocols
[b] difference in frequency due to differences in means and distances for transportation

The urban ACT practice of providing comprehensive direct services cannot be replicated because of the long travel distances involved in serving rural patients. To develop comprehensive plans for each patient, available community resources must be mobilized, trained, and coordinated. When possible, family members or neighbors are engaged in the treatment plan, assisting with administering or delivering daily medication, transporting clients to appointments, and lending support during emergencies.

Since residential and vocational alternatives are more limited in rural areas, independent living and employment do not receive the emphasis found in urban ACT programs. The team does, however, focus on goals related to productive, personally satisfying daytime activities such as hobbies, increased involvement with family, volunteer work, and using available community resources.

The urban ACT practice of a daily team meeting, daily contact with unstable patients, and direct emergency-service availability twenty-four hours per day is impractical in rural areas because of the travel distances involved. Consequently, rural teams meet less frequently and can only be available during a crisis if phone services are available. During regular work days, staff members spend time with support systems, including family members, neighbors, and others to make provisions for potential after-hours crises. The indigenous support persons are educated about alternatives in these instances. Support persons learn that, in addition to contacting the local sheriff, they can contact program personnel in the morning and receive rapid assistance. When clients and their environment are properly evaluated and monitored through regular and consistent home visits during the day, timely interventions can be made and many emergencies avoided.

Community health nurses are ideal rural ACT team members, because they can perform numerous social work functions. On the other hand, social workers and mental health counselors are not licensed to provide essential nursing functions such as administering and monitoring medication. In rural outreach work, nursing job descriptions include traditional social work, vocational rehabilitation, and home health duties.

The numerous administrative responsibilities of staff in their role of "keeper of the medical record" involve managing documentation according to agency requirements (i.e., making sure that consent forms are signed, treatment plans developed, physician's signatures on treatment plans secured, prescriptions signed, services received by the patient documented, billing submitted, etc.). Because of the inordinate amount of travel time involved, these duties are difficult to manage efficiently. Ideally, large sections of the medical records, such as assessment and progress notes, can be dictated by staff during routine travel and transcribed by clerical support staff the following day.

A Rural ACT Program/Case Vignette

One Rural ACT program named Rural Outreach, Advocacy and Direct Services (ROADS) was developed by the Charleston/Dorchester Community Mental Health Center in 1988 and targeted for individuals with severe and persistent mental illness and high utilization of centralized inpatient facilities. The ROADS staff spend most of their time monitoring medication effects and compliance, facilitating access to basic resources, and developing and educating each patient's indigenous community support network about his or her illness and treatment. The team provides financial management and other individualized services, such as the use of sign language for deaf patients; the nature and frequency of staff contacts are determined by each patient's individual needs.

The original ROADS clinical team was comprised of two community health nurses with extensive background in home health care and social work and a part-time psychiatrist. With expanded funding from a substantial federal grant (CMHS research demonstration), the ROADS team has been expanded to include two social workers, two additional registered nurses, and a full-time secretary. On a typical day, ROADS staff travel in teams of two in state-owned vans, carrying a change of clothes, a pair of "mud shoes," a first-aid kit, and other assorted items. Frequently, they get caught in the rain or must trek through a washed-out dirt road. Lunch boxes, fresh water, and a couple of rolls of toilet paper are also essential in the remote rural areas because restaurants and public restrooms are not always conveniently available. In dramatic contrast to a more traditional office-based setting in an urban area, the call of the open road and other characteristics of rural living make rural mental health work especially appealing to this ACT team. The psychiatrist provides direct services for two full days a week and is available by telephone the remainder of the week. The psychiatrist, who is responsible for the pharmacologic treatment and overall clinical status of the clients, visits them in their homes, usually accompanied by another person. The psychiatrist also provides administrative support and education to the team on an ongoing basis (formally in team meetings, informally during work in the field) and supervision of undergraduate and graduate students in the field.

Here is an interesting case serviced by ROADS; it is also featured in the 1994 film *Never too Far* available from Marvin S. Swartz, M.D. at the Division of Social and Community Psychiatry of the Department of Psychiatry at the Duke University Medical Center:

Mr. Martin is a 32-year-old, single, African American male living 45 miles from Charleston on a rural coastal island. We heard about him from neighbors who expressed concern because they had not seen him for several years, although they knew he was still living in his family's home. Suspecting he was mentally ill, they reported the situation to the mental health center. The center's mobile emergency psychiatry team made a home visit and found that he was living in a small, four-room shack with electricity but without running water, toilets, or window screens. He had barricaded himself in one bedroom, wired the door shut, covered the windows, and used a hole in the floor for a toilet. He had previously worked as a farm laborer and socialized with family and friends, but then he became very paranoid. As he explained, he began this self-imposed isolation several years earlier because, "I got into trouble if I came out." He did not bathe and did not change clothes during those years. He always wore several layers of clothing in spite of the intense summer heat and, because of the tightness of his clothing, suffered from impaired circulation in his extremities. He left his room only occasionally at night when no one else was awake. He refused to allow others to enter his room but he accepted food and drink through a partially opened door. As a result of the evaluation he was hospitalized, treated for his paranoid psychosis, and discharged to be followed by the center's ACT team.

He was eventually prescribed an intramuscular long-acting neuroleptic every four weeks and became less paranoid, more communicative, and less isolated. His auditory persecutory hallucinations diminished. The team slowly developed a relationship with Mr. Martin and his family, visiting at least once a week and administering his injections monthly. The team focused on improving his environment and hygiene, arranging through other social services and volunteer agencies for running water in the house, an outhouse, a refrigerator, mattresses, roof repairs, and window screens. They helped him obtain Medicaid and a disability income and worked with his family on basic hygiene and food preparation, including convincing the family not to let their chickens run free in the house. Mr. Martin's environment was problematic, as his alcoholic father had attempted to kill him on four occasions because of his frustration over his son's unwillingness to work. However, Mr. Martin strongly resisted efforts to be relocated, even with other family members who lived nearby, because, as he noted, "This is home and it is the only home I've ever known."

Mr. Martin still lives with his family. He now sits out with his family in the living room and walks around in the yard. He eats with the family and takes baths about weekly, although he still prefers to wear layers of clothes. With medications, he is without any hallucinations and his paranoia is minimal. He and his family appreciate the improvements in their living conditions and the increase in family income.

Homeless Mentally Ill

The growth of homelessness among persons with mental illness since the late 1970s has been proportionately greater than the overall increase in the homeless population. There have been a number of studies of homeless persons with mental illness that provide a profile of their life experiences and clinical characteristics. Reports of these studies provide a description of a population that appears to be seriously mentally ill, severely disabled, and multiply diagnosed, having poor coping skills and entrenched patterns of inability or resistance to engaging with available mental health, health, and social services.

Homelessness among persons with mental illness has been widely characterized as primarily the result of state hospital deinstitutionalization. Careful studies of the homeless mentally ill, however, do not support the notion that deinstitutionalization has been a major factor in the homelessness of the mentally ill. Instead, the evidence points to several other factors: a marked reduction in low-cost housing stock in the United States, primarily as a result of the gentrification of older neighborhoods that had large numbers of low-cost housing units; worsening economic conditions for those lowest on the economic scale; and, as low-cost housing began to decrease, tenants with little support and a diminished capacity to cope, who were the most likely to become homeless. In brief, persons with severe and persistent mental illness were the most vulnerable and, as a result, are overrepresented in the homeless population today.

In 1982, the NIMH was designated to coordinate federal efforts to address the problem of homelessness among persons with mental illness. In response NIMH established an Office of Programs for the Homeless Mentally Ill. However, significant initiatives were not forthcoming until Congress passed the William B. McKinney Homeless Assistance Act in 1987. The McKinney Act funds a homeless mental health services formula grant (PATH) to state mental health agencies and competitive research/demonstration grants. The PATH grants have served as a vehicle for the Office of Programs for the Homeless Mentally Ill to promote a Community Support Systems approach among states organizing homeless services (see Table 4-2, p. 33). Between 1988 and 1990, NIMH also funded 36 research and demonstration projects. The major findings of these projects were the following:

1. Outreach to homeless persons with mental illness must be linked to housing, mental health, and case management services.
2. Intensive case management must be provided on an ongoing basis.
3. Linking clients to mainstream community mental health services is not a viable approach in most communities.
4. Many homeless persons with mental illness have co-occurring substance use disorders and services for both disorders need to be integrated.
5. Residential stability requires intensive, on-site support.
6. Strategies are needed to increase services integration among the multiplicity of agencies and organizations with a role in serving homeless persons within a given geographic area.

In 1993, the Office of Programs for the Homeless Mentally Ill funded a nine-state, eighteen-site research demonstration program specifically focused on the effects of adding services integration strategies to intensive case management services. This five-year, $85-million project will be the primary focus of the Office of Programs for the Homeless Mentally Ill through the end of this century.

ACT Modifications for Homeless Populations

Homeless mentally ill persons tend to be difficult to engage in treatment. Those with co-occuring substance use disorders are particularly difficult to engage and, as a subgroup, tend to exhibit more aggressive, illegal, and self-destructive behaviors. Most estimates of the prevalence of psychoactive substance use among psychiatrically impaired homeless individuals are in excess of 50 percent. These individuals usually deny psychiatric and substance use problems and do not readily submit to the demands of program structure.

One of CMHS's McKinney-funded research projects was designed to measure the effectiveness of ACT for homeless persons with severe mental illness. The Baltimore ACT team made some interesting modifications to the ACT model in order to facilitate their work with homeless persons. One modification of the model in the Baltimore ACT team was the employment of two full-time client advocates who were individuals with a history of homelessness and/or mental illness (advantages to hiring clients as staff are discussed in Chapter 7). The Baltimore ACT team is staffed by approximately twelve full-time-equivalent personnel: a master's level social worker program director, a half-time psychiatrist medical director, a half-time staff psychiatrist, the two consumer advocates, six clinical case managers (two nurses, two social workers, two with other relevant experience), and a project secretary-receptionist. The team also has a family outreach worker under contract from the area NAMI group for ten hours a week and a half-time nurse practitioner trained to treat medical problems.

A second modification is that, while the entire team works with all clients, each person is assigned to a "mini-team" composed of a clinical case manager, a psychiatrist, and a consumer advocate. Thus, rather than operating from a "pure" shared caseload orientation, the six case managers carry individual caseloads and are assisted by the other members of their "mini-team." This modification was based on the premise that engaging a homeless person in treatment is more likely to occur by having only a few of the staff at a time getting to know the client.

A third modification was that services would be discontinued once the treatment plan objectives had been met and clients were stable for a period of time. The type of clients the team has "discharged" from their service are: those with less severe disorders and relatively few previous inpatient admissions for psychotic episodes; those with personality disorders as their principal need for mental health care; and those who, for various reasons, had never been offered or received standard outpatient treatment.

Preliminary results of the Baltimore ACT homeless study indicate that over a one-year period of time the ACT team, as compared to standard services, produced reductions in inpatient hospitalization, increased the use of outpatient services, improved housing outcomes, and decreased symptoms. The Baltimore ACT team continues to function as before, with post-research funding from a variety of state and federal sources.

Use of Street Drugs

A very high percentage of the population of persons with severe mental illness use alcohol and street drugs. Approximately 50 percent of these individuals develop alcohol and/or illicit drug use disorders during their lives. Substance use destabilizes mental illness and interferes with rehabilitation. Among severely mentally ill persons it is associated with symptomatic worsening, violence, living instability, and homelessness. In addition, this group consumes a significant portion of health care expenditures (especially costs associated with hospital-based resources) and other social resources, such as those of the judicial and law enforcement systems.

The use of illicit substances increases the severity of a severely mentally ill client's psychopathological status and, therefore, the intensity of care required. These "dually diagnosed" clients tend to have more complaints and global distress, are less well adjusted, and have poorer outcomes than clients who are not dually diagnosed. They tend to lack motivation for recovery, need long-term care because of frequent relapses, and cannot tolerate the intense emotional confrontation that is often characteristic of traditional substance abuse treatment modalities. Because of these differences, utilization of traditional substance abuse treatment programs for this population is generally unsuccessful.

The growing prevalence of substance abuse and mental illness comorbidity and the high prevalence of multiple behavioral, medical, and other related problems in this population has raised critical policy-level questions concerning the effectiveness of traditional interventions for these individuals. Compounding the problem is the fact that, in most states, mental health service systems and substance abuse treatment systems have remained separate, often functioning in parallel rather than in an integrated fashion. This becomes problematic when dealing with clients who require the best from both systems. Clients easily become lost between the two systems. Moreover, it is not unusual for one of the two systems to extrude a client from their system because of the presence of the other disorder.

It is clear that for optimal results to be obtained an integrated approach is necessary, where treatments for both the mental illness and substance abuse disorder are addressed by the same team of clinicians. Integrated substance abuse mental health treatment can be ideally provided through the assertive community treatment model.

Specific Interventions

1. *Acute detoxification strategies.* These strategies are safe and effective and, through the home-based support of an ACT team, can often be accomplished on an "outpatient" basis. Note that hospital residential treatment programs, which are among the more expensive treatment programs available in the treatment marketplace, have not been established as effective beyond the point of discharge from the hospital. In fact, the modalities with the most evidence of effectiveness in the general substance abuse population are social skills training and brief motivational counseling, which are far less expensive than residential programs.

2. *The use of pharmacological adjuncts.* Strategies that make use of pharmacological adjuncts to psychosocial programs are adding to our knowledge base. Treatments using disulfiram (Antabuse) and methadone are often ranked in the top half for effectiveness among available modalities, as measured by efficacy and costs. The effectiveness of naltrexone as an adjunct to currently available psychosocial interventions has some good preliminary evidence. Double-blind studies of serotonin uptake inhibitors have not, as yet, been conducted.

3. *Strategies that involve well-structured "talking therapies."* These include:
   a. psychoeducational persuasion groups focused on education about dual disorders, enlisting acceptance of prescribed medication to reduce mental and physical discomfort, and developing motivation to become abstinent;
   b. counseling and education to create cognitive dissonance regarding their reasons for using substances and the effects of substance use on their lives; these combine high expectations for abstinence with assurance of ongoing support in the event of relapse;

c. individual psychotherapy from a primary therapist to decrease psychological distress;

d. group therapies focused on symptom control and abstinence through self-management; and

e. relapse education and rapid intervention to prevent relapse in response to stressors.

4. *Social and environmental strategies.* These include: nurturing the development of internal control over symptoms and impulses associated with substance use through positive reinforcement and peer group pressure and support; use of mutual support groups (Double Trouble, GROW, Manic-Depressive, AA, and NA, etc.) both within the agency and in the community; assistance in establishing social relations with other non-using persons and in decreasing amounts of unstructured time; promotion of living arrangements, daytime activities, and social relations with non-using persons; and assistance in getting and keeping employment when abstinence is achieved or substance use has decreased to the point that reliability is likely.

5. *Strategies that employ more coercion and/or external controls.* These include: contingency contracting or written agreements (contracts) between clients and the team, with stated contingency rewards and consequences; random urine and breathalyzer screening; external structure through such means as SSI/SSDI payee status; written agreements between client, probation/parole officer and team, when applicable, with conditions attached to probation and parole in the event of conviction for a crime; and civil commitment.

Assertive Community Treatment and Dually Diagnosed Clients

Integrated substance abuse and mental health treatment in the context of the assertive community treatment model presents several advantages. For example, through utilizing assertive community outreach, problems with compliance and "treatment dropout" are reduced. The ACT team's focus on assisting clients regarding basic needs augments the significance of the therapeutic relationship and provides for greater motivation/leverage for behavioral change. Staff may employ strategies such as using payeeships, guardianships, or legal sanctions as inducements to engage and comply with treatment. Staff can utilize a continuum of supervised living and day treatment settings in which close monitoring can be provided, as needed. Of greatest importance for ACT staff in developing effective strategies for treating dually diagnosed clients is the perspective summarized by Drake in 1997, to "proceed slowly and gently, with a low level of affect, a high level of structure, and attention to psychotic vulnerability."

A four-stage model of treatment, developed by Osher and Kofoed, is helpful in maintaining a long-term perspective and can guide ACT clinicians in planning and deciding what specific interventions are appropriate at a particular point in time:

Stage 1. Engagement. Developing a trusting relationship, or working alliance.
Stage 2. Persuasion. Helping the client to perceive the adverse consequences of substance use in his or her life and to develop motivation for recovery.
Stage 3. Active Treatment. Helping the patient to achieve stable recovery, whether that is controlled use or abstinence.
Stage 4. Relapse Prevention. Helping the client to maintain a stable recovery.

Clients typically cycle back and forth between engagement and persuasion initially and may relapse from active treatment or relapse-prevention stages. Since clients usually don't consider substance use as problematic, insisting on abstinence in the early stages is not useful and may drive them away from treatment. Help with engagement often comes from others, such as family members, public guardians, or the criminal justice system (as a condition of probation, parole, or conditional discharge). Even when they are well engaged in mental health treatment, clients often remain unmotivated with respect to substance abuse treatment, but progress in the persuasion stage can be made during crises and hospitalizations, when the consequences of abuse are more evident. As noted earlier, the clinician's approach must be nonconfrontational, supportive, and empathic.

The "active treatment" strategies include psychoeducational, medical, behavioral, familial, social, and vocational interventions. They are aimed at developing a repertoire of attitudes, skills, and supports used to maintain abstinence. During this phase, numerous setbacks should be expected. Among this group of treatment strategies, behavioral interventions that involve identifying, practicing, and reinforcing specific skills are particularly useful and can be done in a group format.

Recovery should not be expected before a period of years in treatment; so, despite the obvious disappointments caused by setbacks, it is important that staff and families remain nonconfrontational and supportive. Note that the expensive, twenty-eight-day inpatient treatment model has not been demonstrated to be superior to traditional outpatient services for any significant period of time beyond discharge. This long-term perspective regarding recovery is quite compatible with ACT. Once new clients become engaged with staff, it is relatively easy to begin the process of engagement to a substance abuse treatment. In fact, Drake and colleagues assert that, in their extensive work with this population, clients in ACT programs are six times more likely to attend substance abuse treatment than those who are subjected to more traditional substance abuse treatment approaches.

Suggested Readings

Becker, D. R., & Drake, R. E. (1993). *A working life: The Individual Placement and Support (IPS) Program*. Concord, NH: New Hampshire-Dartmouth Psychiatric Research Center.

Bond, G. R. (1992). Vocational rehabilitation. In R. P. Lieberman (Ed.), *Handbook of psychiatric rehabilitation* (pp. 244–275). New York: Macmillan.

Cook, J. A., Razzano, L. A., Straiton, M. D., & Ross, Y. (1994). Cultivation and maintenance of relationships with employers of people with psychiatric disabilities. *Psychosocial Rehabilitation Journal, 17*(3),103–116.

Dixon, L. B., Krauss, N., Kerman, E., et al. (1995). Modifying the PACT model to serve homeless persons with severe mental illness. *Psychiatric Services, 46,* 684–688.

Drake, R. E., McHugo, G. J., Becker, D. R., et al. (1996). The New Hampshire study of supported employment for people with severe mental illness. *Journal of Consulting and Clinical Psychology, 64*(2), 391–399.

Drake, R. E., & Osher, F. C. (1997). Treating substance abuse in patients with severe mental illness. In S. W. Henggeler & A. B. Santos (Eds.), *Innovative approaches for difficult-to-treat populations* (pp. 191–209). Washington: American Psychiatric Press.

Lachance, K. R., Deci, P. A., Santos, A. B., et al. (1997). Rural assertive community treatment: Taking mental health services on the road. In S. W. Henggeler & A. B. Santos (Eds.), *Innovative approaches for difficult-to-treat populations* (pp. 239–252). Washington: American Psychiatric Press.

Mobray, C. T., Leff, S., Warren, R., et al. (1997). Enhancing vocational outcomes for persons with psychiatric disabilities: A new paradigm. In S. W. Henggeler & A. B. Santos (Eds.), *Innovative approaches for difficult-to-treat populations* (pp. 311–348). Washington: American Psychiatric Press.

Osher, F. C., & Kofoed, L. L. (1989). Treatment of patients with both psychiatric and psychoactive substance use disorders. *Hospital & Community Psychiatry, 40,* 1025–1030.

Test, M. A., Knoedler, W. H., & Allness, D. J. (1985). The long-term treatment of young schizophrenics in a community support program: The training in community living model: A decade of experience. *New Directions for Mental Health Services, 26.*

⟫⟩⟩❱ 11 ❰❰❰❰

ACT Financing and Administration

In developing new payment systems, policymakers must choose between targeted strategies that attempt to influence the treatment process directly and those that establish broad goals for effectiveness, access, and efficiency while allowing providers more latitude in the treatment process. These choices profoundly influence how and to whom ACT is available. Nevertheless, different modes of financing and reimbursement contribute to or detract from the effectiveness, accessibility, and efficiency of ACT and changes in these mechanisms will have major implications for further dissemination of ACT Programs.

—Robin Clark, 1997

Essential Administrative Support for ACT

It is absolutely essential to have a supportive administrative environment for ACT clinical services to fully succeed. There are several administrative principles that are essential to the successful development of these programs; these are discussed below.

Philosophical and Instrumental Commitment of Agency Director

The provision of effective ACT services requires more administrative flexibility than is often found in traditional outpatient and residential settings (e.g., flex-time for staff, increased clinical supervision, accountability for outcome). Successful implementation of ACT programs requires staff to adapt to a vari-

131

ety of changes in work routine and shifts in perspectives about their professional role. Starting new programs within existing agencies has been most
effective when the agency heads were firmly committed to a community-
based care system and able to hold staff accountable for adherence to the
model. Changes in agency policies are unlikely without the strong support of
the director. Likewise, a high level of commitment is needed to respond
assertively to complaints from stakeholders, who may be threatened by or at
philosophical odds with a new project.

Facilitating the Recruitment of Staff with the Requisite Characteristics

Agency administrators can facilitate or impede staff recruitment processes. As
mentioned earlier, the personal and interpersonal qualities of the staff represent critical levers for change. Individuals who have experience with a
range of human problems and are sensitive to cultural and ethnic issues are
extremely valuable. Supervisory experience suggests that several staff characteristics are associated with positive treatment outcome, including:

1. a high level of commitment to clients and their families to ameliorating
   their problems;
2. the capacity to identify and focus on individual and family strengths;
3. high intelligence and strong common sense;
4. social and interpersonal flexibility;
5. real world experience and/or being "street wise"; and
6. self-confidence.

Agency administrators who understand and appreciate the ACT system's aims can facilitate the recruitment of new staff and/or the transfer of
ideal staff from existing programs by personally helping to overcome agency
obstacles to the hiring of such individuals.

Providing Sufficient Training and Access to Case Consultation

The difficulty and complexity of treating persons with severe and persistent
mental illnesses require that staff be provided with considerable initial and
continuous training, as well as access to the trainers for case-specific consultations. Despite the fact that many staff have advanced degrees, in general
professional training programs do not include courses in ACT in their curriculum. Therefore, it is important to have access to training dollars specifically for ACT training and consultation. These may include several full days
of intensive training prior to project start-up, intermittent booster training

sessions, consultations via conference calls with ACT experts, and on-site supervision from an ACT expert.

Commitment to Positive Interagency Relations and Coordinated Care

The appeal of ACT is, in part, based on its assumption of accountability as the single point of responsibility for assuring that the broad needs of clients and their families are met and its orientation to treating the individual within the context of his or her family and social system. While the ACT model is considered to be a self-contained system with regard to addressing the clinical, rehabilitation, and case management needs of clients, ACT's success is also dependent on its initiating and maintaining positive relationships with all agencies that share responsibility for serving similar populations of clients. Because of the severity and scope of the problems most clients of ACT programs have, the development of collaborative and coordinated interagency relations is essential. It is critical to brief and seek the support of key stakeholders (mental health, justice, law enforcement, education, social welfare, substance abuse agencies) throughout the process of developing a new program. Each project (or, if the project is part of a larger agency, the parent agency) should have a community advisory board with family, neighborhood, and agency representation. On an ongoing basis, a percentage of project staff time is explicitly devoted to the development and maintenance of positive interagency relations.

Public Policy and Financial Support

A primary reason for the incomplete dissemination of ACT throughout the United States is the inertia of the existing systems of community and hospital care. Financing streams, which have both shaped and been shaped by the historical emphasis on hospital and office-based care, have not been altered to facilitate and thus promote the provision of ACT-based care. No third parties provide specific coverage for ACT. Only under Medicaid can a portion of the cost of ACT be recouped through the insurance mechanism. Even for Medicaid-covered populations, the considerable start-up costs of launching an ACT program, combined with the state share of Medicaid expenditures, represent barriers to state mental health agencies interested in its development. Although Medicaid has modified its rules so that it covers some ACT practices, it is essentially a fee-for-service arrangement and does not cover many crucial ACT services. The financial strategy that best fits an ACT model is one where the program is funded using a modified capitated system, for example, an ACT program would be funded to provide services for a hundred clients. The staff would then be able to do whatever was necessary to help the client without having their activities shaped by whether what they did was a reimbursable service.

Broad dissemination of ACT within a state cannot occur without the support of the state agencies responsible for the care of the populations targeted. The broad dissemination of ACT in several states has been the result of the recognition of its effectiveness by the state-level human service directors, who have initiated policies and incentives to spur statewide development. New and reallocated state funds have been directed toward the development of ACT programs and Medicaid coverage (for which the majority of individuals in need of these services are eligible) has been specifically tailored to the program models. The opportunity to reallocate state funds results from the success of ACT in preventing expensive institutional placements. By the middle of the 1980s, sufficient numbers of ACT programs had been developed in several states to accrue substantial budgetary savings from the reduced use of more expensive modalities. Entire service delivery systems have been transformed in those states that were allowed to reallocate the savings to further expand the availability of ACT services. It is no coincidence that the majority of states rated as having exemplary state mental health systems as described in the 1990 Public Citizen Report have developed ACT programs on a wide scale. Third-party payers would be wise to decrease reimbursement for expensive, restrictive, and unproven treatments and increase support for more clinically efficacious and cost-effective alternatives. ACT holds great promise for accomplishing a shift from the inappropriate dominance of the hospital in the health-care system to community-based programs.

Cost of ACT: You Get What You Pay For

In order for a program to successfully achieve its specific objectives for its clients, the staff must be perfectly clear about what they are trying to accomplish. While this may seem obvious, it is not unusual to find individual clinicians who, when asked what they are trying to accomplish, are less than clear about their goals with the client, the program's goals for its caseload, and the goals of the sponsoring agency and its rationale in facilitating financing for the program. Clarity of purpose is good for team functioning; it facilitates reaching desired outcomes and helps maintain good staff morale.

By design, ACT programs currently in existence in the United States vary with regard to their objectives. In order to simplify communications the rationale should be clear to all stakeholders. For example, if competitive employment is not a direct program objective (i.e., the expected outcome of direct interventions that are given a high priority within the program and encouraged in the team's daily work) the administrators of the program should make this clear to all parties involved (rather than hiding the fact or feeling guilty about not being in philosophical synchrony with the current thinking in the Madison flagship PACT model). Reaching certain targets often requires strong, coordinated team efforts, and the success of well coordinated teamwork depends on the level to which its objectives can be clarified and measured. Teams that are not clear about their objectives will have a more difficult time achieving outcomes that can be said to have occurred as a direct result of their services.

The desired outcomes of programs based on the original PACT model, as outlined by Test in 1992, are:

1. Reduced symptomatology and reduced subjective distress
2. Increased community tenure
3. Enhanced satisfaction with life
4. Improved psychosocial functioning

Clearly, some of these outcomes are easier to measure than others. For example, increased community tenure is reflected both by a reduced number of hospitalizations and shortened lengths of hospital stay, as well as a reduced number of changes in residential settings over a given time interval. It is not surprising, therefore, that community tenure is the one outcome domain most consistently reported by ACT programs as a measure of their success. It is often unclear what other outcomes are directly sought by many programs in operation, since much less quantifiable information about other outcome domains is usually reported. Our assumption is that most programs have difficulty measuring their accomplishments in the psychosocial functioning and quality of life domains and so are not able to report these results in a clear and convincing manner.

Further clarification of program objectives at the level of local ACT teams is warranted. For instance, should a team addressing Test's first desired outcome (reduced symptomatology and subjective stress) be required to provide effective substance abuse treatments? Should the program be required to provide the newer, more effective medications that have fewer side effects but are significantly more expensive? If so, at what agency level should these decisions be made? What financial mechanisms can be put in place to integrate expensive new treatments as they appear in the marketplace?

Similarly, if a program endorses striving to achieve the third and fourth desired outcomes (enhanced satisfaction with life and improved psychosocial functioning), should it be required to provide supported employment services? Clearly, the intent of these desired outcomes implies striving toward facilitating a normal daily routine, including competitive employment, and the "gold-standard" programs will target outcomes that involve effective vocational rehabilitation (as well as state-of-the-art substance abuse treatments).

Despite the argument that a client cannot be said to have reached full community integration without gainful employment, in reality this is not an aim of most programs in operation. In some of these programs, the administrators acknowledge up-front that, in their opinion, it is not cost-effective to strive for employment as an outcome of mental health treatment programs; consequently, they do not expect (and may discourage) competitive employment as a principal program objective and domain for the daily work of the staff. This, combined with the fact that clinicians have traditionally considered these clients' potential for competitive employment to be low, makes competitive employment a particularly difficult outcome to achieve on a wider scale. The vast majority of mental health programs and providers do not recognize employment services as one of their core functions. Only in a very limited number of states do certification standards require that treatment teams include vocational specialists; nevertheless, *a significant percentage of clients of mental health services say they want to work.*

The financial implications of clarifying these questions are significant. An ACT program for a hundred clients, available around the clock, seven days a week, can be supported at a cost of approximately $7,000 to $8,000 per year per client. At this level of funding, it is possible to offer services designed to achieve clinical stabilization, low use of hospitals, long community tenure, progressive stability in housing, and assistance with management of finances. However, this level of support is not sufficient to support the additional vocational specialists and substance abuse specialists needed for a high percentage of clients to achieve successful outcomes regarding competitive employment and freedom from the influence of alcohol and other psychoactive substance abuse.

Among states that have undertaken statewide or large-scale development of ACT programs, average annual per client expenditures range from $5,000 to $18,000, varying primarily based on the size of the team, the staff's level of professional education, the ratio of clients to staff, the use of additional team members as vocational specialists and substance abuse specialists, and whether the particular setting requires staff to be available around the clock, seven days a week for direct service provision. In community mental health centers without ACT programs, the average per client expenditure for usual services is reported in the range of $2,000 to $3,000. Thus, providing ACT would represent at least a doubling of the average outpatient treatment expenditure per client for those clients chosen to be cared for by the service; however, this difference would be more than made up through the reduction in costs of hospital services.

Financing the start-up costs of ACT can pose a challenge. Cost analyses in controlled studies of ACT have demonstrated ACT to be less costly than usual services only when expenditures for hospital treatment are factored into the analyses. Thus, financing for large-scale development of ACT programs could potentially be offset by reductions in expenditures for hospital care in both state and community hospitals. Without strategic systematic reform, however, "savings" from reduced use of one sector does not necessarily result in an actual shift of resources to expand a preferred mode of care in another sector. The recent momentum at the federal and state levels to stem the growth of health-care expenditures while expanding health insurance coverage may lead to increased focus on the cost containment potential of ACT. It is unfortunate that, in this era of budget reductions and health-care cost-cutting, we have a paucity of well established mechanisms for monitoring client outcomes.

ACT program financing is further complicated by the fact that, rather than a single form of treatment, ACT is a combination of health and social services delivered efficiently. This "mix" of services can be problematic for some states. Nevertheless, there are now several states that have developed financial strategies leading to successful implementation of ACT programs designed to meet specific objectives.

As an example, administrators in New Hampshire, recognizing that higher payments for office-based treatment would limit the growth of ACT programs, changed their method of paying for Medicaid case management services to include a special category called Mental Illness Management Services (MIMS). MIMS pays mental health centers, specifically, for services delivered outside of traditional treatment settings; case management services had formerly been reimbursed with an all-inclusive monthly rate. The new payment system is a mix of retrospective and prospective payment. Centers receive a smaller monthly payment to cover indirect services like advocacy and service coordination, plus a variable amount based on the number of MIMS service units delivered.

In Connecticut, where ACT program development start-up funds originally came from federal and foundation grants, new teams continue to be established in the absence of new funding. As the state hospitals have downsized, staff have voluntarily transferred to community programs to promote the creation of new ACT teams. In addition, state-operated programs and private, nonprofit community agencies have combined staff to create new teams, overcoming numerous obstacles, such as resistance from unions and problems created by differing benefit packages (i.e., staff performing same jobs might have different vacation benefits, or some would get extra pay for carrying on-call pagers and others not). The state has also invited competitive proposals for new team development with financial support for start-up costs at the level of $150,000 per year for two years.

In Michigan (which has the most ACT teams in operation), the process involved careful study of needs, delineation of desired outcomes, the establishment of demonstration projects used to publicize advantages of the model, and gaining the support of legislators, clients, advocacy groups, and providers. Michigan's first twenty teams were funded through expansion funds provided by the state legislature. The state's Medicaid procedures were initially not well suited for ACT and with the help of the state manager of Medicaid (the Michigan Department of Social Services), a new service was created, under the Psychosocial Rehabilitation Option, called Assertive Community Treatment. Noteworthy was the fact that the Medicaid rules were adjusted to fit the model instead of making the model fit Medicaid. Additional resources were freed up because ACT reduced inpatient expenses and those saved hospital dollars were reallocated to community-based programs. This was possible because Michigan's funding strategy provides community mental health boards with a single budget to purchase both community-based and hospital-based services, and thus money not spent for hospital use is available for community services. This strategy was so successful that it was also used to develop and finance field-based service teams for youth and elderly populations.

Given these considerations, it is important for administrators to decide, right from the beginning, on the number of clients to be served and the desired outcomes. This will allow projections about the number and types of staff to be hired (i.e., how much to spend, on whom, and for what purpose). To this end, we recommend the following practical guidelines for considering the relationship of desired outcomes, team size, staff backgrounds, and caseload size:

1. In order to achieve only reduced symptomatology, reduced subjective distress, and increased community tenure (fewer hospitalizations) of severely mentally ill clients with low levels of substance use, a minimum of one staff person per twelve clients will be necessary (i.e., a team composed of ten clinicians can achieve these outcomes with a caseload of one hundred twenty

clients). Staff backgrounds necessary to achieve these outcomes are medicine, nursing, social work, and other generalist clinicians needed to fill out the staff (psychologists, mental health counselors, etc.). We want to stress that the above outcomes, which do not include a special effort to help clients get competitive jobs and do not require a strong substance abuse treatment effort, are minimally acceptable.

2. In order to achieve the same outcomes as above with clients with a higher level of substance use, a minimum of one staff person per ten clients will be necessary (i.e., a team composed of ten clinicians can achieve these outcomes with a caseload of a hundred clients). Staff backgrounds necessary to achieve these outcomes are medicine, nursing, social work, plus staff trained in substance abuse treatment, as well as other generalist clinicians needed to fill out the staff (psychologists, mental health counselors, etc.).

3. In order to achieve the above outcomes plus improved psychosocial functioning, enhanced satisfaction with life, and competitive employment, a minimum of one staff person per eight clients will be necessary (i.e., a team composed of ten clinicians can achieve these outcomes with a caseload of eighty clients). Staff backgrounds necessary to achieve these outcomes are medicine, nursing, social work, substance abuse specialist, and vocational specialist, as well as other generalist clinicians needed to fill out the staff (psychologists, mental health counselors, etc.). For optimal outcomes to be achieved, there should be a half-time psychiatrist, a full-time substance abuse specialist, and a full-time vocational specialist for every fifty clients.

These client-to-staff ratios do not include administrative support personnel, the all-important secretary/receptionist being one of them. The type and number of administrative support staff will vary from state to state, depending on billing and credentialing requirements. They will also vary from program to program, depending on the continuum of possible administrative contexts, from stand-alone programs to those that are part of large agencies. Finally, remember that the intake rate needs to be low enough to maintain a stable service environment—no more than five or six per month as the team develops.

Current Controversies for Program Administrators

In terms of operating an ACT team, there are two interrelated issues that are usually debated prior to program start-up and often require administrative guidance and policy clarification. The first has to do with the proper population of clients that ACT should serve. There is usually agreement that the

population served should be persons with severe and persistent mental illness; the debate is about whether this means all or just a subpopulation of
them. The second but related debate has to do with how long the client
should stay in an ACT program. Those who take the position that all persons
with severe and persistent mental illness should be managed by an ACT team
also argue that the client should stay in the program for as long as he or she
needs any mental health treatment. On the other hand, those who take the
position that ACT teams should be reserved for only the most difficult-to-
manage clients in the system also argue that once the difficult-to-manage
client has been well stabilized, as evidenced by at least one year of not
requiring emergency services or the hospital, the client could be gradually
transitioned to less intensive programing, such as a clubhouse or medication clinic. Although there is a paucity of data at the present time to guide
us in these two areas, these issues are critically important and are therefore
worthy of discussion.

To have an ACT team serve all clients who have a severe and persistent
mental illness for as long as they need any treatment certainly ensures continuity and integration of services; however, it raises the problem of having the
team carry more and more clients as new clients are admitted to the service.
The advocates of this plan propose a solution to this logistical problem of an
increasing client-to-staff ratio: They propose that when the ACT team has too
many clients, it split into two teams. The new team, managing the stabilized
clients, will be able to operate with a lower client-to-staff ratio. However, this
solution requires, as new difficult-to-treat clients are admitted, new funds to
bring each team up to the appropriate staff level.

Those who argue that ACT should specialize in the difficult-to-manage
client and that stabilized ACT clients should be transitioned to other, less intensive programs, contend that this is a cost-effective way for a system to manage
all the persons in that system with severe and persistent mental illness. They
argue that, as clients are gradually transitioned to programs of lesser intensity,
many clients will eventually be assigned to programs that have a client-to-staff
ratio of a hundred-to-one. They maintain that, in a program of that size, clients
would be naturally leaving—through death, moving away, or recovery—at the
same rate that clients would be coming into the program; thus, costs would not
be constantly rising. Although there is no research evidence that bears on this
question, they maintain that there are programs in the country that are successfully operating this way. They also point out that other programs that have
a different primary focus from ACT (such as a clubhouse, which is oriented
almost entirely towards rehabilitation with a strong ethic of client empower-

ment) may be more useful to stable clients than an ACT program. Again, at present there are no data to inform us on this question. We need research on the characteristics of mentally ill individuals within various program models to determine which aspects of client functioning are associated with different program settings. Such information would be useful for matching particular clients with specific program types. Matching could ensure optimal availability of the most intensive services for people with the greatest need and would facilitate the allocation of services in a more efficient and judicious manner. Finally, the feasibility and wisdom of moving stable clients from more to less intensive service models is another critical question deserving research.

From a systems perspective, an enormously important concern is the cost of the service per client. It would be extremely useful if one could assign clients to the most economical service necessary to help them achieve the goal of living a stable life of decent quality in the community. The Dane County, Wisconsin, system has been operating with ACT teams, as well as with other models for working with persons with severe and persistent mental illness, for almost two decades. In this system, there are various types of continuous care programs that specialize in working with subpopulations of the seriously mentally ill, based on difficulty to treat. These programs vary in composition and working schedules, accordingly. The most difficult to treat clients are served by ACT teams that are mobile, have a ten-to-one client-to-staff ratio, and operate seven days a week, with a cost of approximately $8,000 per client per year. Very stable clients are assigned to teams of psychiatrists and nurses; here, the client is seen in the office, the client-to-staff ratio is close to a hundred-to-one, and availability is weekdays during normal working hours, with a cost of just over $1,000 per client per year. Finally, clients who fall between these two groups in difficulty to treat are assigned to the clubhouse, which is patterned after the Fountain House model. The client-to-staff ratio is approximately twenty-to-one, the client comes to the clubhouse for services, and the clubhouse is open seven days a week, at a cost of about $4,000 per client per year. In a system like this it is critical, during client evaluation, to determine the kinds of clinical services that a particular client needs and how to identify the program or programs in the system that can best provide those services. Grouping clients by diagnosis, or even by the overall severity of their illness, is less useful when making these decisions than is focusing on the specific service needs of individual clients.

The Dane County system uses a typology that allows clinicians to think about clients on a number of different dimensions. Seven characteristics—willingness to come in for services, medication compliance, need for structured daily activities, ability to self-monitor, frequency of crises, need for professional psychological support, and degree of case management services required—are directly related to the kind of programming that each client requires in order to live successfully in the community. The ACT programs in Dane County are assigned clients who, on the items noted above, would require assertive, mobile, and intensive services that are available twenty-four hours a day. The authors of this volume recommend using this typology in determining which clients in their system require an ACT team. The typology is described in more detail below.

Willingness to come in for services. Clients vary in their willingness to come in for services. Some come to all their appointments, some are unwilling to come in at all, and others are unpredictably variable and frequently miss appointments. In many communities around the country, clients falling into the latter two categories are called "unmotivated" or "treatment resistant" and are not treated until they become sick enough to qualify for involuntary hospitalization. We believe that approach reflects poor clinical judgment; we contend that an unwillingness to come in for services by persons with severe and persistent mental illness is a manifestation of the illness and thus requires a specialized response.

Medication compliance. Clients who respond to medications but are not willing to take them reliably require a treatment approach that includes very careful monitoring and the use of a wide variety of incentives, augmented by legal coercions when necessary, to ensure that they take needed medication.

Need for structured daily activities. Many clients in the system have a social network of their own or a way of adequately structuring their own time and do not require a professional team to provide structured daily activities. However, other clients require special help in structuring their daily activities.

Ability to monitor oneself. Clients who can recognize that an increase in irrational thoughts and hallucinations is a signal that their disease is getting worse and that they should seek help can be treated by a program that provides less intensive follow-up than clients who are less able to monitor themselves. Those clients who have not yet learned to monitor themselves often interpret their irrational thoughts and hallucinations as a signal that they are in personal danger and respond by staying in their room and discontinuing their normal social and treatment contacts. They often become isolated and withdrawn and, if not intensively followed, emerge only when their symptoms become very overt.

Frequency of crises. Clients who have frequent or severe crises need treatment from a program equipped to provide intensive and extensive crisis intervention and resolution services. Clients who have few crises do not need such a program.

Need for professional psychological support. Some persons with severe and persistent mental illness have a well-established folk network that gives them a sufficient amount of psychological support to maintain stability. Many, however, require professional psychological support in order to maintain stability. These clients require more intensive services.

Degree of case management services required. Some clients are able to negotiate complicated social and bureaucratic systems well enough and do not require much specialized case management services. Others require help in everything from budgeting money to shopping for food. Again, the intensity and the cost of services vary according to individual needs.

A Final Note of Warning to Administrators

We have learned that administrators trained in traditional treatment models may have difficulty understanding the conceptual framework that drives ACT treatment and may not be able to grasp the advantages of field-oriented service delivery models. Some look at such a drastic paradigm shift with a great deal of suspicion. Others shy away from it simply because they do not want to take the heat for insisting their staff see clients in their natural surroundings rather than in their offices. It is not unusual to find administrators who purposely create obstacles to ACT program implementation.

We are in the midst of revolutionary changes in the structure of the health-care delivery system. Like political revolutions, the new regime may be no better or, perhaps, worse than the former. We are already witnessing never before heard of developments in the structure of service systems, such as hiring private firms to manage public sector mental health funds. Administrators should keep in mind that while the public mental health sector in the United States has traditionally provided both clinical and social services to the population for which it is responsible, private insurers and managed care firms have not. Private insurers and managed care firms traditionally have not assumed the responsibility of addressing the deterioration in social functioning caused by a person's mental illness. They operate under a medical model that conceptually liberates them from responsibilities in this domain and allows them to focus strictly on medical treatments. They usually support intensive services only to the degree that they are required to alleviate acute symptoms of a disease. Thus, beware of contracts with the private sector to care for public-sector clients; they will likely lead to lower levels of psychosocial outcomes than your current system.

Unfortunately, since we, as a field, have not been able to reach a working consensus on all the treatment objectives (desired outcomes) of ACT, we often do not speak in a united voice. In addition, we don't routinely use, in our clinical settings, measures of client "well-being" (i.e., role functioning and quality of life); thus, we would have no way of knowing if the kinds of social goals advocated in this book were sacrificed by these companies in the name of cost savings. For example, we already know of instances where state public mental health authorities have contracted out mental health services to private companies who, in their desire to hold down costs, have heavily used the very same centralized state hospital facilities that we have been trying to move away from. After all, the cost of a night of care at a centralized state hospital is around $200-$300, compared with the cost of a night at a community hospital, which can range anywhere from $400 to over $1,000 a night. This is obviously a good business decision and likely to be praised by shareholders. However, just as obviously, it is a poor clinical decision, as it removes clients from their home communities and deprives them of the continuity of care available to them if hospitalized on the psychiatric ward of their community hospital. Finally, note also that the private sector has very limited experience with non-hospital crisis stabilization alternatives; therefore, you shouldn't expect much of an interest from them in creating these options.

In closing, administrators who emphasize outcomes congruent with those desired by clients and their families will likely steer clear of danger in these changing times. A persistent focus on outcomes, rather than staff satisfaction or the bottom-line cost figures, will encourage the growth of models that produce the best results for clients.

Suggested Readings

Clark, R. E. (in press). Financing assertive community treatment. *Administration and Policy in Mental Health.*

Essock, S. M., & Kontos, N. (1995). Implementing assertive community treatment teams. *Psychiatric Services, 46,* 679–683.

Meisler, N., Detrick, A., & Tremper, R. (1995). Statewide dissemination of the training in community living program. *Administration and Policy in Mental Health, 23*(1), 71–76.

Meisler, N., & Santos, A. B. (1996). Case management of persons with schizophrenia and other severe mental illnesses in the USA. In M. Moscarelli, A. Rupp, & N. Sartorius (Eds.), *The handbook of mental health economics and health policy: Vol. I. Schizophrenia* (pp. 179–194). West Sussex, England: Wiley.

Meisler, N., & Gonzales, M. C. (1997). Medicaid financing. In S. W. Henggeler & A. B. Santos (Eds.), *Innovative approaches for difficult-to-treat populations* (pp. 395–410). Washington: American Psychiatric Press.

Mobray, C. T., Collins, M. E., Plum, T. B., et al. (in press). The development and evaluation of the first PACT replication. *Administration and Policy in Mental Health.*

Mobray, C. T., Plum, T. B., & Masterson, T. (in press). Harbinger II: Deployment and evolution of assertive community treatment in Michigan. *Administration and Policy in Mental Health.*

Plum, T. B. (1997). Statewide program dissemination in Michigan. In S. W. Henggeler & A. B. Santos (Eds.), *Innovative approaches for difficult-to-treat populations* (pp. 411–421). Washington: American Psychiatric Press.

Stein, L. I. (1989). Wisconsin's system of mental health financing. *New Directions for Mental Health Services, 43,* 29–41.

Torrey, E. F., Erdman, K., Wolfe, S. M., et al. (1990). *Care of the seriously mentally ill: A rating of state programs* (3rd ed.). Washington: Public Citizen Health Research Group and National Alliance for the Mentally Ill.

Appendix

Introduction

The forms in this appendix were developed by the Mental Health Center of Dane County, Inc. (MHCDC). The public mental health system in Dane County, Wisconsin, has earned an international reputation for its comprehensive and integrated system for serving persons with severe and persistent mental illness. Through a variety of programs, the MHCDC provides most of the services in this county for this population. Included among these services are the Center's five ACT teams, each using forms similar to the ones in this book; the forms in this book are the ones being used by the Center's Gateway ACT Team.

The forms included in the appendix are The Initial Assessment and Plan, which is used to develop the initial treatment plan as soon as possible after the client is admitted to the program, and the fifteen assessment forms utilized to collect information for the development of the comprehensive treatment plan, which should be completed within one month of the client's admission to the program. Although the teams use additional forms, such as consent forms, money management forms, etc., they were not included in the book because they were too site specific and of limited usefulness.

INITIAL ASSESSMENT AND PLAN

Name_____ Admission Date_____

Diagnosis:

      Axis I _____

      Axis II _____

Functional Impairment (check and describe):

☐ Vocational_____

☐ Educational _____

☐ Homemaking _____

☐ Social/Interpersonal_____

☐ Community Integration_____

☐ ADL's_____

Initial Plan:

_____

_____

_____

_____

_____

_____

_____

This individual evidences a need for CSP care and CSP services are medically necessary in this case.

_____
Psychiatrist   Date

_____
Team Leader   Date

_____
Client   Date

PSYCHIATRIC FUNCTIONING AND HISTORY INTERVIEW FORM

Client name _____

Date(s) of interview(s) _____

_____

Interviewers _____

_____

Current Psychiatrist _____

_____

Current Medications and Dosage

_____

_____

_____

See attached sheet for additional meds

Medication compliant? Y / N If not, specify:

_____

_____

_____

_____

_____

_____

Do you take medication independently? Y / N If no, give specifics regarding where meds are dispensed, frequency of deliveries, office pickups:

_____

_____

_____

_____

_____

_____

_____

Mental Health Center of Dane County, Inc.

May be reproduced

_____

_____

_____

_____

Do you attend psychiatric appointments willingly/regularly? Y / N If no, why not?

_____

_____

_____

_____

_____

If yes, how often?

_____

_____

Do you remember the onset of your illness? Y / N Specify age, place, circumstances, who affected, how treated, client's perceptions then and now:

_____

_____

_____

_____

_____

_____

_____

_____

_____

_____

_____

_____

Have you received education regarding your mental illness? Y /N Explain:

_____

_____

_____

_____

_____

_____

Would you like more information? Y / N

How does your mental illness make you feel?

_____

_____

_____

What is your understanding of your own mental illness?

_____

_____

_____

_____

What is your perception of the treatment and support you have received for your mental illness? What seemed to work and what didn't?

_____

_____

_____

_____

_____

_____

_____

_____

How do your symptoms interfere with your daily functioning? Specify symptoms, frequency, specific ADLs affected:

_____

_____

_____

_____

_____

_____

_____

_____

_____

_____

_____

_____

Do you have any med preferences, what's worked in past, what differential side effects have you experienced, what's changed and why has it changed?

_____

_____

_____

_____

_____

_____

_____

_____

_____

PRESENTING PSYCHIATRIC SYMPTOMS

Symptoms	Self-Report	Interviewer	Reports of Others
Delusions			
Paranoia			
Grandiosity			
Thought			
insertion			
withdrawal			
Somatic			
Special Powers			
Persecutory			
Nihilistic			

Symptoms	Self-Report	Interviewer	Reports of Others
Affect			
Apathetic			
Euphoric			
Angry			
Blunted			
Broad			
Flat			
Constricted			
Sad			
Happy			
Inappropriate			
Silly			
Anxious			
Speech			
Normal			
Pressured			
Tangential			
Mute			
Incoherent			
Circumstantial			
Blocking			
Perseveration			
Flight of ideas			
Hallucinations			
Auditory			
Visual			
Gustatory			
Tactile			

Symptoms	Self-Report	Interviewer	Reports of Others
Thought Content			
Obsessions			
Compulsions			
Phobias			
Ideas of reference			
Poverty of			
thought content			
Sexual preoccupation			
Religious preoccupation			
Suicidality			
Homicidality			
Worthlessness			
Hopelessness			
Magical thinking			
Other			
Irritability			
Impulsivity			
Silliness			
Passivity			
Manipulative			
Demanding			
Negativistic			
Suspiciousness			
Rigidity			
Dramatic			
Narcissistic			
Mood			
Depressed			
Angry			
Anxious			
Irritable			
Expansive			
Fearful			
Sad			
Euphoric			
Happy			
Sarcastic			
Pessimistic			

Symptoms	Self-Report	Interviewer	Reports of Others
Motor Status			
Slouches			
Erect			
Tremors			
Stooped			
Hyperactive			
Restless			
Other Symptoms			

Please give brief description, including frequency of symptoms, which distinguishes client from others:

Hallucinations:

Delusions:

Other bizarre thought content/behaviors:

_____

_____

_____

_____

_____

Have you ever been hospitalized? Y / N If yes, where/when?

Hospital	Date

Have you ever lived in an institution? Y / N If yes, where/when?

_____

_____

_____

_____

_____

_____

(Complete records to be sent for, see Record of Hospitalizations)

How do you think the CSP can help you?

_____

_____

_____

_____

_____

What do you do when you experience hallucinations? (How do you feel; how do you cope?)

_____

_____

_____

_____

_____

How do you deal with delusions/paranoia?

_____

_____

_____

_____

_____

Have you ever felt like hurting yourself? Y / N Did you ever act on these feelings? Y / N Specify when/how/who was involved:

_____

_____

_____

_____

_____

_____

_____

_____

_____

Have you ever felt suicidal? Y / N Threatened suicide? Y / N
Attempted suicide? Y / N Specify (identify all incidents of suicide attempts if possible):

_____

_____

_____

_____

_____

_____

Have you ever felt like hurting someone else? Acted on those feelings? Y / N Specify:

_____

_____

_____

_____

Have you ever damaged property unintentionally?

_____ Hurts others (when and under what circumstances)

_____ Destroys property (when and under what circumstances)

_____ Yells, screams, swears

_____ Throws things

Additional interviewer observations/comments:

_____

_____

_____

_____

_____

When you need assistance managing behavior, the things that are most helpful are:

_____ Being comforted   _____ Change of environment

_____ Being ignored   _____ Physical redirection

_____ Verbal redirection   _____ Rewarding a different behavior

Additional interviewer observations/comments:

_____

_____

_____

_____

_____

Have you been sexually or physically abused by others? (when, duration, circumstances, perpetrators). What happened? Have you talked to anyone about it? If yes, did that help? If no, would you find it helpful to talk to someone about it?

_____

_____

_____

_____

_____

_____

_____

_____

_____

_____

_____

_____

_____

Interviewers:

If possible, have the client assist you in completing the record of hospitalizations and institutionalizations. When this interview is completed, furnish a copy to the clinical coordinator and arrange for the client to have a mental status examination with the clinical coordinator. The mental status exam is required as part of the in-depth assessment.

PSYCHIATRIC HOSPITALIZATION RECORD

(Complete this form for each hospitalization)

Client_____ Hospital_____

Admission Date_____ Discharge Date_____

Symptoms/circumstances few months prior to admission (med regime, med compliance, stressors, over-all functioning, etc.):

_____

_____

Symptoms/circumstances weeks prior to admission (include above):

_____

_____

Presentation at and stated need for admission (appearance, symptoms, prognosis, any legal involve-ment, etc.):

_____

_____

Medications while in hospital:

_____

Hospital course (include treatment milieu, significant behavior and symptoms, response to treatment):

_____

_____

Discharge diagnosis_____

Discharge medications_____

Discharge disposition (include prognosis, DIC plans, etc.):

_____

_____

_____

HEALTH HISTORY

Date _____

Name _____ D.O.B. _____

City _____ Birthplace _____

Age _____ Allergies _____

Ethnic: C   B   A   H   NA

Present illness(es) _____

I. CLIENT PROFILE

A. CURRENT LIFE SITUATION

Name of: 1. Internist_____Clinic_____

2. Psychiatrist_____Clinic_____

3. Eye doctor _____Clinic_____

4. Dentist _____Clinic_____

B. OCCUPATIONAL HEALTH

1. Any physical condition that may affect performance on the job site?

_____ back   _____ eyesight

_____ knee   _____ hearing

_____ dizziness   _____ seizures

_____ fear of heights

2. Have you had an injury while at work? Describe:

_____

_____

3. What odors, smells, or fumes bother you?

_____

_____

C. NUTRITIONAL CARE INFORMATION SHEET

1. Previous Diet counseling:

   Kind of diet/s _____

   Rec'd. individual diet info. Y / N

   Desires printed diet information Y / N

   Tried to lose/gain weight Y / N

Physical Data:

Height _____

Present weight _____

Desired weight _____

Ideal weight _____

Max. weight _____

Min. weight _____

2. Factors influencing food intake:

   Has good appetite Y / N

   Has elimination problems Y / N

   Follows three-meal pattern daily Y / N

   Has food allergies Y / N

   Eats at normal pace Y / N

   Has cravings for sweets/fried/salty Y / N

   Is a smoker Y / N

   Has other cravings Y / N

3. Typical daily intake:

_____

4. How many times a week do you have a meal at a fast food restaurant? _____

D. SLEEPING HABITS

1. Going to sleep:

   _____ average nightly hours of sleep

   _____ difficulty falling asleep

   _____ trouble staying asleep

2. Waking up:

   _____ waking up often during the night

   _____ early morning awakening

   _____ feel rested when you wake up

   _____ tired during the day

II. HEALTH HISTORY

A. GENERAL HEALTH INFORMATION

1. Any specific health problems or concerns you would like to discuss?

_____

B. PAST HEALTH HISTORY

1. When was your last PE? _____

2. When was your last chest x-ray? _____

3. Date of last pelvic exam? Pap Smear results? Were you asked to report yearly?

_____

4. Date of last dental exam? What kind of dental work has been done?

_____

5. Date of last eye exam? Do you wear glasses or contacts? For distance or reading?

_____

6. Date of last hearing exam? Results? _____

7. Has anyone ever shown you how to do a breast self-exam? _____

8. Have you ever received information on testicular self-exam? _____

C. CHILDHOOD HEALTH

1. Did you have a regular family doctor? _____

2. Do you remember or know if you had: (+ = yes, 0 = no)

_____ chicken pox   _____ mumps

_____ tonsils removed   _____ measles (if known what type?)

_____ strep throat   _____ rheumatic fever

_____ scarlet fever

3. Do you know if you've been immunized for: (+ = yes, 0 = no)

_____ rubella or measles   _____ polio (vaccine/oral)

_____ tetanus   _____ influenza

_____ TB skin test

result:_____

D. ADULT HEALTH

1. Medical illnesses, e.g., pneumonia or ulcers. Explain:

_____

_____

_____

_____

_____

2. Surgeries or medical hospitalizations. Explain:

_____

_____

_____

_____

_____

3. Transfusions. Explain:

_____

_____

_____

_____

_____

4. Serious injuries/accidents. Explain:

_____

_____

_____

_____

_____

5. Medications (include over-the-counter)

Name	Dosage	Frequency	Reason for Taking

III. BIRTH CONTROL/SEXUALLY TRANSMITTED DISEASE

A. BIRTH CONTROL

1. Are you, or have you ever been, sexually active?

2. Do you use birth control? If not, why? Do you know where to go for that information?

3. If you have had sexual intercourse, how often do you or your partner use any kind of the following:

_____	the pill	_____	IUD
_____	time of the month (natural)	_____	withdrawal
_____	condom (rubber)	_____	foams or gels
_____	diaphragm	_____	no birth control
_____	sponge	_____	other

4. Have you ever been pregnant or fathered a child? Give details:

_____

5. Do you want any information about birth control? _____

B. SEXUALLY TRANSMITTED DISEASE*

1. Have you ever had a sexually transmitted disease (V.D.) such as:

_____	syphilis	_____	herpes
_____	gonorrhea	_____	chlamydia
_____	vaginitis	_____	other

Describe _____

_____

2. Have you ever had symptoms of:

_____	burning urination	Males:	
_____	white or yellow discharge	_____	drip from penis
_____	abdominal pain	_____	pain from scrotum
_____	sores around genital area	_____	sore on penis

3. Do you know if your partner has had symptoms of a sexually transmitted disease?_____

4. Do you want more information about sexually transmitted disease? _____

5. Would you like information about sexuality? _____

*Inform that the greater the number of sexual partners a person has, the higher the risk of getting a sexually transmitted disease.

IV. FAMILY HISTORY

A. HEALTH OF BIOLOGICAL PARENTS:

__ diabetes	__ allergies	__ scoliosis	__ hyperactivity
__ high blood pressure	__ heart disease	__ back problems	__ obesity
__ cancer	__ arthritis	__ sickle cell anemia	__ thyroid

V. CURRENT HEALTH STATUS

Date of Review_____

A. Describe your general health (include specific goals client would like to work on):

_____

_____

B. Specific review

1. Eyes: Visual aides, itching, diplopia, tearing, pain, blurring.

_____

2. Throat: Soreness, difficulty swallowing, lumps.

_____

3. Head: Describe any incident/history of head injuries or headaches.

_____

4. Ears: Describe any ear problems (ringing, wax build-up, earaches, frequent infections, difficulty hearing).

_____

5. Nose: Describe any nose problems (sinus problems, nosebleeds, frequent colds).

_____

6. Teeth: When do you brush your teeth? hard or soft brush? dental floss? mouthwash? gums bleed? cavities? toothaches?

_____

7. Lungs: Have you ever experienced any of the following: wheezing? blood (in sputum)? night sweats? sputum color? coughing? asthma? pneumonia? bronchitis? shortness of breath? other?

_____

8. Heart: Have you ever been told that you have high blood pressure? Do you have chest pains? racing heart? swelling of feet? blue nails/lips?

_____

9. Breast: Do you have any breast lumps or discharge from the nipple? pain/tenderness? biopsy? mammogram? fibrocystic disease?

_____

10. GI: Do you ever have any loss of appetite? nausea & vomiting? diarrhea? ulcers? constipation? pain in stomach? black stools? blood in stools? chalky stools?

_____

How often to you have a bowel movement?_____

11. GU: Do you need to get up in the night to urinate? blood in urine? trouble starting/stopping flow? bladder/kidney infections? burning?

_____

How often do you urinate? _____

12. GYN: Menses/Age of onset _____

    Amount of flow _____

    Intermenstrual bleeding _____

    Pain_____

    Itching/Irritation_____

    Menopause_____

    Last pelvic exam_____

    Results_____

    Pregnancies_____

    Live Births _____

    Abortions_____

13. Musculoskeletal: How long can you stand before legs, back, neck, joints start to hurt?

_____

14. Neuro: Have you ever had a seizure? Describe:

_____

    Fainting spells? Describe:

_____

    Tremors? Describe:

_____

15. Blood: Do you bruise easily?_____

    Have you ever been told you were anemic?_____

16. Endocrine: Do you have fluctuating weight? Describe:

_____

Do you have diabetes?

      increased urination

      increased appetite

      increased thirst

      weight loss

      ever have blood sugar level tested

17. Skin: Do you have any rashes? excessive dryness or oiliness? sores near mouth or reproductive organs?

_____

How often do you bathe? _____

18. Physical exam _____

  A. General Appearance_____

    _____

  B. Vital Signs _____

     P _____

     T _____

     R _____

     B/P   (R)_____(L)_____

19. Additional interviewer observations/comments _____

_____

_____

_____

_____

Reviewer _____ Date _____

ALCOHOL AND DRUG ASSESSMENT

Client name _____ Date of interview_____

Interviewer(s) _____

Do you use alcohol or other drugs? Y / N If yes, please describe usage, including average daily or weekly consumption of alcohol or other drugs:

_____

_____

_____

_____

_____

_____

_____

_____

_____

Have you ever used alcohol or drugs in the past? Y /N If yes, please describe usage and types of drugs:

_____

_____

_____

_____

_____

_____

_____

_____

_____

Do your family or friends have concerns about your drug and/or alcohol use? Y / N

_____

_____

_____

_____

_____

Are you able to stop drinking or using other drugs when you want to? Y / N

_____

_____

_____

_____

_____

Have you ever or do you currently attend AA or NA? Y / N If yes, when? If yes, do you have a sponsor?

_____

_____

_____

_____

_____

Have you gotten into fights or other trouble when drinking? Y / N Describe:

_____

_____

_____

_____

_____

Have you ever been arrested when you have been drinking or using drugs? If yes, please describe, including time and events:

_____

_____

Are you aware of possible interaction between your prescribed medications and illicit drugs or alcohol? Y / N If yes, please describe:

_____

_____

Have you gotten into trouble at work due to drug or alcohol use? Y / N If yes, when?

_____

_____

_____

_____

_____

_____

_____

_____

Have you ever received treatment for AODA issues? Y / N If yes, when and where? Outcome?

_____

_____

_____

_____

_____

_____

Does anyone in your family have AODA issues? Y / N If yes, who, and were they ever treated? Please give specific dates and where treatment occurred if possible:

_____

_____

_____

_____

_____

_____

_____

If yes, do you or have you ever attended Al-Anon meetings?

_____

Have you ever been in detox? Y / N If yes, when?

_____

_____

_____

_____

_____

_____

Have you ever been arrested for drunk driving? Y / N If yes, please give specifics:

_____

_____

Do you smoke? Y / N Chew tobacco? Y / N If yes, what amounts?

_____

Do you drink coffee? Y / N Soda pop? Y / N If yes, in what amounts? Does it interfere with sleep? Y / N

_____

_____

_____

_____

_____

_____

_____

ACTIVITIES OF DAILY LIVING INTERVIEW FORM

Client name_____Date(s) of interview(s)_____

Interviewer(s)_____

Food and Nutrition Skills:

Refrigeration and cooking facilities available in residence? Y / N If no, how does resident prepare food?

_____

_____

_____

Typical day's diet*:

    Breakfast:

    Lunch:

    Supper:

    Snacks:

Special dietary needs? Y / N If yes, identify:

_____

_____

Purchases variety of foods from all food groups? Y / N

Excessive consumption of sweets/junk food? Y / N

*Use space in additional comments to include disparities between client report and others' observations.

MEAL PLANNING/PREPARATION

Activity	Independent	With Prompts	With Supervision	Unable to Accomplish
Grocery Shopping				
Plans meals in advance				
Understands nutrition				
Applies nutritional principles				
Makes out shopping list				
Can prepare cold meal				
Can prepare hot meal				
Can use recipe to prepare meal				
Can use standard range				
Food intake appropriate to nutritional needs				
Can use microwave oven				

Additional interviewer observations/comments:

_____

_____

_____

_____

_____

_____

MAINTENANCE/HOUSEKEEPING SKILLS

Activity	Independent	With Prompts	With Supervision	Unable to Accomplish
Cleans kitchen				
Cleans bedroom				
Cleans livingroom				
Cleans bathroom				
Purchases cleaning supplies				
Uses washer				
Uses dryer				
Keeps dirty and clean clothes separated				
Stores clean clothes properly				
Does hand washing				
Does simple mending				
Vacuums				
Dusts				
Empties trash				
Identifies repair/maintenance needs				

Does client have or would client be willing to use cleaning service?

Additional interviewer observations/comments:

_____

_____

_____

_____

PERSONAL HYGIENE/GROOMING SKILLS

Activity	Independent	With Prompts	With Supervision	Unable to Accomplish
Brushes teeth				
Wears clean clothing				
Does laundry				
Has personal hygiene items (toothpaste, deodorant)				
Free of body odor				
Trims nails				
Shaves or trims facial hair				
Combs hair				
Washes hair				
Bathes or showers				
Uses deodorant				
Does menstrual cares				
Wears makeup appropriately				

Incontinent Y / N Bowel Y / N Bladder Y / N

Frequency:

If yes, have you seen your physician regarding incontinence? Y / N If yes, is there a medical etiology involved? If you have not seen your physician, why not?

_____

_____

Purchases/wears Depends independently/needs reminder

_____

_____

Does client have unusual grooming habits? Y / N Identify:

_____

_____

_____

Does anyone currently provide assistance in ADLs? Y / N Who? When? How often?

_____

_____

_____

Additional interviewer observations/comments:

_____

_____

_____

_____

_____

MOBILITY SKILLS

Transportation:

Walks Y / N

Uses Bus Y / N

Car Y / N

Cab Y / N

Bike Y / N

Motorcycle Y / N

Subway or other mass transit Y / N

Do you use special transportation?

_____

_____

_____

Do you make your own transportation arrangements? Y / N If not, who does and why?

_____

_____

_____

Do you have a driver's license? Y / N

Personal mobility:

Physical limitations impairing mobility Y / N

Describe:

_____

_____

_____

_____Ambulates independently

_____Needs aid for ambulation

_____Wheelchair _____Electric _____Manual _____Needs assistance

_____Crutches, cane, walker   _____Short distances only

_____Needs supervision/assist with stairs _____Cannot use stairs

Uses public transportation Y / N

Crosses streets safely Y / N

Has adequate sense of direction Y / N

Can arrange transportation Y / N

Knows way around residence Y / N

Drives car Y / N

Knows way around neighborhood Y / N

Additional interviewer observations/comments:

_____

_____

_____

_____

RECREATION/LEISURE SKILLS

Hobbies _____

Leisure activities	**Y / N**	**Frequency/Circumstances**
Television		_____
Movies		_____
Restaurants		_____
Music		_____
Participation in sports		_____
Socializing with friend		_____
Other		_____

RRC	Y / N	How often?_____
Yahara House	Y / N	How often?_____
CLIP Program	Y / N	How often?_____
Off the Square Club	Y / N	How often?_____
Other clubs	Y / N	How often?_____

Additional interviewer observations/comments:

_____

_____

_____

_____

SOCIAL SKILLS

Can begin interaction with another person Y / N

Has a reciprocal friendship Y / N

Comfortable interacting with unfamiliar people Y / N

Shows concern for others Y / N

Enjoys spending time with others Y / N

Prefers to spend time alone Y / N

Needs assistance of others to maintain relationships Y / N

Describes self as shy Y / N

Describes self as outgoing Y / N

Additional interviewer observations/comments:

_____

_____

_____

_____

_____

_____

_____

COMMUNICATION

Method(s) of communication:

Sign language Y / N

Oral Y / N

Can communicate need to others Y / N

Can initiate conversation Y / N

Can follow 1-step direction Y / N

Can follow 3-step directions Y / N

Can use telephone Y / N

Needs assistance using telephone Y / N (check areas of needed assistance):

_____ Answer telephone _____ Dial telephone _____ Find telephone number

Additional interviewer observations/comments:

_____

_____

_____

_____

_____

INTERPERSONAL RELATIONSHIPS

Marital Status:

Number of casual friends (identify by name):

_____

_____

_____

Close friends (identify by name):

_____

_____

_____

Length of friendships:

_____

_____

Describe status of relationships and frequency of contact with friends:

_____

_____

_____

Frequency of contacts with family:

   Parents _____

   Siblings _____

   Children _____

Describe nature of relationships:

_____

_____

Do you argue with family/friends? Y / N How frequently? Specify:

_____

_____

Additional interviewer observations/comments:

_____

_____

_____

_____

MONEY MANAGEMENT, BANKING

Activity	Independent	With Prompts	With Supervision	Unable to Accomplish
Understands function of money				
Can use a calculator to determine change				
Can determine change due after a purchase				
Maintains a savings account				
Maintains a checking account				
Pays monthly bills				
Can understand a bank statement				
Manages day-to-day purchases				
Comparison shops				

Additional interviewer observations/comments:

_____

_____

_____

TIME MANAGEMENT

Usually keeps appointments Y / N

Makes it to work/daily activities, etc., on time Y / N

Able to structure time independently Y / N

Typical daily schedule:

_____

_____

Additional interviewer observations/comments:

_____

_____

_____

PROBLEM-SOLVING AND DECISION-MAKING

How do you go about making decisions for yourself?

_____

_____

_____

What do you take into consideration when you make a decisions?

_____

_____

_____

Give an example of a good decision you have made and why you think it was a good decision:

_____

_____

_____

Additional interviewer observations/comments:

_____

_____

_____

_____

SAFETY SKILLS

Do you have a working smoke detector? Y / N

What would you do if there was a fire in your home?

_____

_____

_____

Do you know how to extinguish a grease fire? Y / N Describe:

_____

_____

_____

Give an example of a medical emergency:

_____

_____

_____

What would you do in a medical emergency?

_____

_____

_____

Have you been the victim of an assault by a stranger? Y / N If yes, please describe:

_____

_____

_____

Have you been the victim of an assault by someone you know? Y / N If yes, please describe:

_____

_____

_____

Have you been the victim of a property crime? Y / N If yes, please describe:

_____

_____

_____

Do you walk alone at night? Y / N

Do you lock your apt. door when home? Y / N

Do you lock your apt. door when gone? Y / N

Adequate traffic skills? Y / N

If no, explain:

_____

_____

If you smoke, do you ever smoke in bed? Y / N

Have you accidentally started a fire with smoking materials? Y / N

_____

_____

Do you burn holes in clothing? Y / N

    in furniture? Y / N

    in carpet? Y / N

    many/few? Specify:

_____

_____

Have you ever acted in a way that was dangerous to yourself? Y / N Specify:

_____

_____

_____

Additional interviewer observations/comments:

_____

_____

_____

CULTUROLOGICAL HISTORY

Name_____ Date_____

Interviewer(s) name_____

I. CROSS CULTURAL DIFFERENCES

1. Discuss cultural differences with the client. Begin by pointing out some of the differences you have with the client (e.g., race, religion, ethnicity, socioeconomic class, sex, sexual orientation, etc.). Ask, "Is there anything about me or my background you'd like to know more about?" Then ask, "Do you think our differences will cause any problems, or is there anything about yourself you think I may not understand or appreciate because I'm a European American male, Latina, etc.)?

_____

_____

_____

2. Do you have any ideas about how we might overcome these potential problems?

_____

_____

_____

3. Have you ever been in a (cross cultural) counseling situation before? What were the circumstances? Was that comfortable for you? What made it comfortable/uncomfortable?

_____

_____

_____

4. Do you have any suggestions about how we might provide services in a way that takes your culture into account? How can we provide services to you in a way that is culturally acceptable to you?

_____

_____

_____

II. CULTURE

A. Culture of Origin and Ethnicity

1. Tell me about your ethnic background. (If necessary, model for the client by describing your own ethnic background.)

_____

_____

2. Where did your mother and father come from/grow up?

  Mother (Name:) _____

  Father (Name:) _____

3. Where did your grandparents come from/grow up?

  Mother's Mother (Name:) _____

  Mother's Father (Name:) _____

  Father's Mother (Name:) _____

  Father's Father (Name:) _____

4. How many generations ago did your family/ancestors come to the U.S.?

  Mother's Ancestors _____

  Father's Ancestors _____

5. Why did your family/ancestors leave their homeland?

_____

_____

6. How does that affect you now and your view of your life?

_____

_____

_____

_____

7. Who raised you?

_____

_____

8. Where were you raised?

_____

_____

9. Who was the head(s) of your family (or made the rules in your family)?

_____

_____

10. Who in your community, outside of your family, had some influence on you?

_____

_____

11. Who had the most status in the community you grew up in?

_____

_____

12. How did you fit in when you were growing up (at school, with family and friends, etc.)?

School _____

_____

Family _____

_____

13. Do you relate to the culture you were born into?

_____

_____

_____

_____

14. Is there another culture you see yourself relating to more? Why?

_____

_____

_____

15. Does this present any problems for you?

_____

_____

_____

16. What are your culture's expectations of what it means to be a woman/man? Are you comfortable with fitting/not fitting that expected role?

_____

_____

_____

B. Current Culture/Community

1. Who would you include in defining your family now?

Name and relationship _____

Name and relationship _____

Name and relationship _____

Name and relationship _____

Name and relationship _____

2. Describe your current community or support system:

_____

_____

_____

_____

3. Is there an organization or individual in your community to whom you could go to for help?

_____

_____

4. How does your community view those with a mental illness? How do they view treatment with medications?

_____

_____

5. Who has the most status in your community now?

_____

_____

6. Who are your heroes/heroines? Why?

_____

_____

7. What kind of music/movies/books/TV shows do you like?

Music_____

Movies_____

TV shows _____

Books _____

8. What do you do for fun (sports, crafts, arts, etc.)?

_____

_____

_____

_____

_____

C. Religious/Spiritual Beliefs and Values

1. What religious or spiritual beliefs were you raised with?

_____

_____

2. What were the beliefs of your parental figures (people who raised you)? Did they have the same beliefs (if there was more than one parental figure)? If they didn't, was there conflict?

_____

_____

3. Did you attend services when you were growing up? If so, what churches, temples, synagogues, cathedrals, etc., did you attend and how often?

_____

_____

4. What are your beliefs now? Do you have any particular spiritual or religious beliefs that provide support for you?

_____

_____

5. Do you attend services now? If so, where and how often? If not, would you like to start attending services? If so, where? Could we be of any assistance with connecting you to a congregation?

_____

_____

6. Are there any special practices you observe because of your religious/spiritual beliefs that might be important for me to know about (e.g., special diets, important days of celebration, sweat lodges, etc.)?

_____

_____

_____

7. Do you have any religious/spiritual beliefs that influence how you view mental illness or medication?

_____

_____

8. Is there any tension between your religious/spiritual beliefs and your behavior/lifestyle (e.g., your sexuality, chemical use, etc.)? Between the beliefs you were raised with and your behavior/lifestyle?

_____

_____

D. Language (Clarify unfamiliar terms, e.g., clinical terminology, cultural or generational slang, used by either client or therapist.)

1. What do you prefer to be called?

_____

2. Are you offended by any specific words/terms?

_____

_____

3. What is your communication style (e.g., lots of gestures/body language, rapid loud speech, high context vs. low context communication style)?

_____

_____

4. What language do you speak at home? What language do you prefer to communicate in? Will it be a problem for you to communicate in the language of the therapist?

_____

_____

_____

E. Social, Economic, Environmental, and Political Factors

1. Describe the neighborhood you grew up in. What did it look like, sound like, smell like, feel like? Would you describe it as a wealthy, middle-class, working-class, or poor community?

_____

_____

How did/does this affect you?

_____

_____

2. How did you perceive your parents' (or parental figures') status? Was your parents' status different from your friends' parents' status?

_____

_____

Was your parents' status different from the community or neighborhood you lived in?

_____

_____

3. What is your status now compared to your parents' status? Is your status different than your parents' status when they were your age?

_____

_____

4. Where are you compared to the friends you grew up with?

_____

_____

5. We live in a society which often attributes personal value to monetary success. Does this affect your self-concept? How?

_____

_____

6. Are you involved in the political process in any way? Are you aware of current legislation about areas that affect you?

_____

_____

III. VALUES OF THE CLIENT AND THE CLIENT'S COMMUNITY VIS-À-VIS MENTAL ILLNESS AND TREATMENT

1. How does your community view mental illness (e.g., is it all right to tell people in your community that you have a mental illness or is it best to keep this a secret)?

_____

_____

2. What do people in your community generally view as the cause of mental illness (e.g., a difficult childhood, biochemical, environmental stress, etc.)?

_____

_____

3. What is the generally accepted form of help for your problem from your community's point of view?

_____

_____

4. What is the generally accepted view in your community about the use of medications to treat mental health problems?

_____

_____

5. What would your friends say about your being here today asking for help?

_____

_____

6. Would you be embarrassed to tell family members or friends that you came for help today? (How accepting is the community?)

_____

_____

7. If your son, daughter, brother, sister, etc., had this kind of problem, what would you recommend that he or she do?

_____

_____

8. What do you think causes mental illness?

_____

_____

9. What do you think caused your problems?

_____

_____

10. How do you feel about the use of medications to treat your problems?

_____

_____

11. How have you dealt with this problem before? (What are your coping mechanisms?)

_____

_____

12. How has your community intervened before with regard to this problem?

_____

_____

13. Is there any way that your community might be helpful to you now?

_____

_____

IV. PROBLEMS THAT STEM FROM RACISM OR BIAS IN OTHERS

1. Begin this discussion by demonstrating your understanding of how the mainstream culture oppresses people from the client's culture (e.g., an African American exhibiting the symptoms of a mental illness is more likely to be arrested and jailed than taken to a hospital for treatment, etc.). Once the idea is established, ask, "Have you ever experienced prejudice, stigma, or negative reactions directed toward you because of your culture, race, gender, sexual orientation, etc.?"

_____

_____

_____

_____

_____

_____

2. Have you ever experienced prejudice because of being diagnosed with a mental illness, or have people related to you negatively because they know you are receiving treatment for a mental illness?

_____

_____

_____

3. How have you dealt with these negative reactions?

_____

_____

_____

4. Is there anything we can do to help minimize the stigma associated with receiving treatment?

_____

_____

_____

ASSESSMENT INTERVIEW: FAMILY/PERSONAL RELATIONSHIPS

Client name_____

Interview date_____Interviewer(s) _____

DOB_____

Are you S/M/D/W?_____

Spouse/Significant Other's name _____

Are you currently involved in a serious relationship? Y / N If yes, specify:

_____

_____

_____

If no, have you had a serious relationship(s) in the past? Y / N Please describe:

_____

_____

_____

Do you have any children? Y / N If yes:

Name	Age	M/S/D	Occupation	Residence

Do you have custody/visitation of minor children? Specify:

_____

_____

_____

Where were you born? _____

Where did you live when you were growing up? List all places, dates, reasons for move:

_____

_____

_____

_____

_____

_____

Parents' names and ages:

_____   _____

_____   _____

Stepparents?

_____   _____

_____   _____

If one or both or your parents are deceased, specify cause of death, date:

_____

_____

Where did your parents grow up?

_____

_____

Parents' occupations:

_____

_____

Siblings?

Name	Age	Occupation	M/S/D	Children	Residence

How did your parents discipline you?

_____

_____

_____

_____

Did your mother and father discipline you in different ways? Y / N Specify:

_____

_____

_____

Were either or both or your parents abusive/assaultive toward you (verbally, emotionally, physically, sexually)? Y / N Specify:

_____

_____

_____

Were any of your siblings abusive/assaultive toward you (verbally, emotionally, physically, sexually)?
Y / N Specify:

_____

_____

_____

_____

_____

_____

Have you ever been abusive/assaultive toward any family member or significant person in your life
(verbally, emotionally, physically, sexually)? Y / N If yes, specify:

_____

_____

_____

_____

How often do you see your parents?

_____

_____

Who initiates contact?

_____

_____

How often do you see your siblings?

Sibling	Frequency of contact	Who initiates contact

Which sibling(s) do you feel closest to?

_____

_____

Do you discuss your mental illness and treatment with your family? Y / N If not, why not?

_____

_____

_____

Are any of your family members familiar with or part of the Alliance for the Mentally Ill? Y / N Specify:

_____

_____

What was it like growing up in your house?

_____

_____

_____

_____

_____

How would you describe your childhood?

_____

_____

_____

_____

_____

What would you like to have been different?

_____

_____

_____

_____

_____

_____

Does anyone else in your family (immediate and extended) have mental health problems? Y / N If yes, specify who and treatment:

_____

_____

_____

_____

_____

_____

_____

Does anyone in your family (immediate and extended) have AODA problems? If yes, specify who and treatment:

_____

_____

_____

_____

_____

_____

_____

Does anyone in your family have serious health problems? Y / N If yes, specify:

_____

_____

_____

_____

_____

How would you describe your relationship with your parents?

_____

_____

_____

_____

_____

Would you be agreeable to having family members involved in your treatment in some way? Y / N If yes, which members and how much and what kind of involvement?

_____

_____

_____

_____

_____

If not, why not?

_____

_____

_____

_____

_____

Would you be interested in having family members or other persons who are significant to you informed about our program and services you receive, even if they are not actively involved? Y / N If yes, specify which members:

_____

_____

_____

_____

If not, why not?

_____

_____

_____

_____

What other family members are important to you (aunts/uncles, grandparents, cousins, etc.)?

Name	Age	Relationship/Occupation	Frequency of contact	Who initiates contact

What unique talents do you possess?

_____

_____

_____

_____

What are your strengths and weaknesses?

_____

_____

_____

_____

How has mental illness affected your life?

_____

_____

_____

_____

Additional/anecdotal information:

_____

_____

_____

_____

_____

ASSESSMENT INTERVIEW: INFORMAL/FORMAL SUPPORTS

Client name _____ Date_____

Interviewer(s) name _____

Informal Supports

Friends:

_____

_____

_____

Family:

_____

_____

_____

Significant Others:

_____

_____

_____

Whom do you contact when you are having a difficult time?

_____

_____

Whom do you contact when you want to share something happy?

_____

_____

Whom do you feel close to?

_____

_____

_____

Do you go to church? Y / N Which? How often?

_____

_____

_____

Do you consider your spirituality to be a support to you during hard times? Y / N

_____

_____

_____

Do you attend a 12-step program? Which one? How often do you attend?

_____

_____

_____

Do you belong to any clubs/organizations? Y / N If yes, specify:

_____

_____

_____

Formal Supports (current involvement):

_____

_____

_____

Agencies

Agency/Service Provider_____

Start Date_____

Primary Contact_____

Services Provided:

_____

_____

_____

Agency/Service Provider_____

Start Date_____

Primary Contact_____

Services Provided:

_____

_____

_____

Agency/Service Provider_____

Start Date_____

Primary Contact_____

Services Provided:

_____

_____

_____

FINANCIAL INFORMATION

Name_____ Date_____

Income Sources (Check all that apply, include amounts if known)

	I	SSI	SSI-E	SSDI	VA Benefits	Earnings	Food Stamps
Amount							

Insurance

_____ Medical Assistance   _____ Medicare   _____ Private Insurance

_____ Life Insurance   _____ Burial Trust   (Specify amount)

Assets (describe and include estimated value):

_____

_____

Other Benefits:

Homestead Credit in last year? Y / N If yes, how much?

_____

_____

If no, why not?

_____

_____

Energy Assistance? Y / N How much?

_____

_____

If no, why not?

_____

Budgeting:

Representative payee? Y / N If yes, give name, address, phone number:

_____

FINANCIAL

Savings account? Y / N Where _____

Checking account? Y / N Where _____

Cosignature required? Y / N _____

CSP Account? Y / N _____

Manages own money? Y / N CSP assistance? Y / N Describe:

_____

_____

_____

_____

Spending money spent on:

_____

_____

_____

_____

Spends money impulsively? Y / N

_____

_____

_____

_____

Willing to budget with assistance? Y / N / None needed. If no, explain:

_____

_____

_____

_____

FINANCIAL

Pays bills with assistance? Y / N / None needed. If no, explain:

_____

_____

_____

_____

_____

Describe current monthly budget:

Rent _____

_____

Utilities _____

_____

Food _____

_____

Telephone _____

_____

Additional interviewer observations/comments:

_____

_____

_____

_____

_____

Person completing this interview _____

Date completed _____

RESIDENTIAL HISTORY

Client name _____ Date of Interview _____

Interviewer(s) _____

Living situations since adulthood:

    Apartment Y / N

    Group home Y / N

    Adult family home Y / N

    Institution Y / N

    Correctional facility Y / N

    Homeless shelter Y / N

    Battered women's shelter Y / N

    Rooming house Y / N

    YMCA/YWCA Y / N

    College dorm Y / N

    With family Y / N

    Own house Y / N

    Short-term care Y / N

    Crisis home Y / N

    Trailer home Y / N

Current address _____

_____

Move-in Date _____ Amount of Rent _____

Subsidized? Y / N

Are you on waiting lists for subsidized housing? Y / N

Have you ever been evicted? Y / N If yes, when and why?

_____

_____

_____

Have you ever done damage to your residences? Y / N If yes, explain:

_____

_____

_____

_____

Have you ever had your security deposit withheld? Y / N If yes, do you know why?

_____

_____

_____

_____

Have you ever experienced discrimination when seeking/maintaining housing? Y / N If yes, explain:

_____

_____

_____

Have you ever let persons not on the lease stay at your place of residence? Y / N If yes, has this been a problem? Y / N Explain:

_____

_____

_____

Is it hard for you to say "no" when others ask if they can stay with you even when they are not on your lease? Y / N

_____

_____

_____

_____

Have the police ever been called to any of your residences? Y / N If yes, explain:

_____

_____

_____

_____

_____

Do you prefer living alone or in a shared living arrangement? Elaborate:

_____

_____

_____

_____

_____

Do you smoke? Y / N Do you prefer living with a smoker/nonsmoker?

_____

_____

_____

_____

What major problems have led to residential moves (evictions, long-term hospitalizations, legal issues, poor apt. maintenance, etc.)?

_____

_____

_____

_____

_____

Past Residences

Move-in/out dates_____

Address_____

Type of residence_____

Alone or roommate_____

Condition of apartment_____

Problems while at apartment_____

Reason for leaving_____

Other comments:

_____

_____

_____

_____

Move-in/out dates_____

Address_____

Type of residence_____

Alone or roommate_____

Condition of apartment_____

Problems while at apartment_____

Reason for leaving_____

Other comments:

_____

_____

_____

_____

Move-in/out dates_____

Address_____

Type of residence_____

Alone or roommate_____

Condition of apartment_____

Problems while at apartment_____

Reason for leaving_____

Other comments:

_____

_____

_____

Move-in/out dates_____

Address_____

Type of residence_____

Alone or roommate_____

Condition of apartment_____

Problems while at apartment_____

Reason for leaving_____

Other comments:

_____

_____

_____

_____

Use additional sheet to describe additional living arrangements

VOCATIONAL PROFILE

Name_____Date_____

Disability_____

_____

Medications/Medical Consideration_____

_____

Financial and/or Medical Benefits_____

_____

1. Mobility Level

_____ Independent (car, walk, public transit)

_____ Requires assistance

_____ Total assistance

Comments:

_____

_____

_____

_____

2. Endurance Level: able to work: ___1-2 hrs.   ___2-4 hrs.

___4-6 hrs.   ___6-8 hrs.

Comments:

_____

_____

_____

_____

3. Ability to Initiate Activities

_____Independent

_____Requires some assistance

_____Total assistance

Comments:

_____

_____

4. Communication Skills

_____Verbal

_____Written

_____Sign language

_____Nonverbal

Comments:

_____

_____

5. Get Along with Co-workers/Peers

_____Does well with others

_____Occasionally has difficulties

_____Has difficulty getting along with others

Comments:

_____

_____

6. Ability to Accept Criticism

_____Yes

_____Sometimes

_____No

Comments:

_____

_____

7. Work Quality

_____Does well

_____Requires assistance

_____Total assistance/unaware of standards

Comments:

_____

_____

_____

8. Work Quantity

_____Work produced at competitive rate

_____Work produced at 1/2 of competitive standards

_____Work produced at less than 1/2 of standards

Comments:

_____

_____

_____

9. Motivation

_____Highly interested

_____Semi-interested

_____No observable expressed interest

Comments:

_____

_____

_____

10. Hygiene and Appearance

_____Acceptable

_____Marginally acceptable

_____Unacceptable

Comments:

_____

_____

_____

11. Support Systems

_____Family

_____Friends

_____Advocate

_____Caregivers

_____Guardian

_____None

Comments:

_____

_____

_____

12. Functional Reading

_____None

_____Sight words/simple reading

_____Fluent

Comments:

_____

_____

_____

13. Functional Math

_____None

_____Count

_____Add/subtract

_____Complex computation

Comments:

_____

_____

_____

14. Time Awareness

_____None

_____Can tell breaks/lunch

_____Aware of minutes/hours

Comments:

_____

_____

_____

15. Attendance

_____Needs daily prompts to attend work

_____Occasional prompts needed

_____Independent attendance

Comments:

_____

_____

_____

16. Emotions

_____Intense emotional swings

_____Apathy

_____Flat affect

_____Typical emotional expression

Comments:

_____

_____

_____

17. Symptoms

_____Active hallucinations

_____Active delusions

_____Disorganized thought

_____Paranoia

Comments:

_____

_____

_____

18. Effect of Disability on Work Environment:

_____

_____

_____

19. Learning Style:

_____

_____

_____

20. Vocational Interests:

_____

_____

_____

_____

21. Educational History:

_____

_____

_____

_____

22. Effect of Work Environment on Symptoms:

_____

_____

_____

_____

22. Vocational History (start with most recent employer)

Name of Employer	Dates	Work Performed	Pay	Reason for Leaving

Name of Person Completing this Interview _____

Date Completed _____

ASSESSMENT: LEGAL INVOLVEMENT

Client_____ Date_____

Involuntary Services_____

Have you ever been involuntarily detained in a hospital or institution (explain if necessary)? Y / N
If yes, what do you recall about the process?

_____

_____

_____

_____

_____

Dates (from, to)_____

Admitted to_____

Presenting problems/behaviors:

_____

_____

_____

_____

Dates (from, to)_____

Admitted to_____

Presenting problems/behaviors:

_____

_____

_____

_____

Dates (from, to) _____

Admitted to _____

Presenting problems/behaviors:

_____

_____

_____

_____

Do you have a guardian? Y / N Dating from _____

If yes, full/limited? If limited, specify (e.g., meds only):

_____

_____

_____

If you do not presently have a guardian, have you had one in the past? Y / N Explain (dates, rationale, type):

_____

_____

Guardian's name _____

How often do you see or have contact with your guardian?

_____

_____

Do you have a representative payee? If yes, who and why?

_____

_____

_____

Law Enforcement

Have you ever been arrested? Y /N If yes, specify (give dates, charges, circumstances for each arrest):

_____

_____

_____

_____

_____

Have you ever been incarcerated? Y / N If yes, specify (starting and end dates, where incarcerated, for what charges, include forensic hospitalizations):

_____

_____

_____

_____

_____

Have you been involved with the police in any other way (police calls for suicide threats, attempts, acting out behavior)? Y / N If yes, specify:

_____

_____

_____

_____

_____

Other legal involvement (eviction proceedings, suits, etc.):

_____

_____

_____

_____

_____

_____

_____

Have you ever been on probation/parole? Y / N Specify (dates, for what charges, where, circumstances):

_____

_____

_____

_____

_____

_____

_____

_____

Are you presently on probation or parole? Y / N If yes, explain reason for parole/probation:

PO's name_____Probation/parole end date_____

_____

_____

_____

_____

_____

_____

Explain reason for parole/probation:

_____

_____

_____

_____

_____

_____

Rules of current probation parole:

_____

_____

_____

_____

_____

_____

Additional interviewer observations/comments:

_____

_____

_____

_____

_____

_____

_____

Interviewer(s) _____

Date _____

AGENCY INTERVIEW FORM

Client name _____ Date _____

Name of agency _____

Staff person interviewed _____

Primary contact person _____

Dates of service: Start _____ Stop _____

Service provided:

_____

_____

_____

_____

_____

Client's schedule:

_____

_____

_____

_____

_____

Client's current involvement (i.e., issues pertinent to attendance, cooperation, attitude, abilities, activities, tasks, etc.):

_____

_____

_____

_____

_____

Client's past involvement (address same issues as above):

_____

_____

_____

_____

_____

_____

Agency's subjective assessment of client's strengths and weaknesses:

_____

_____

_____

_____

_____

Agency description of symptomatology/behaviors while at their program (include how these behaviors specifically affect client's ability to participate in program):

_____

_____

_____

_____

_____

_____

_____

_____

Agency's and client's current goals in agency program:

_____

_____

_____

_____

_____

_____

Agency's opinion about how the CSP could assist client and how agency and the CSP could interface to coordinate and provide consistent services for client:

_____

_____

_____

_____

_____

_____

Additional interviewer observations/comments:

_____

_____

_____

_____

_____

_____

Name of person completing this interview _____

Date _____

FEEDBACK

Please use this sheet to note any problems with the interview instrument or any suggestions you have for improving it, as well as comments about your experience in administering it.

Sequencing of questions:

_____

_____

Clarity of questions:

_____

_____

Difficulty clients have in answering questions (which questions and why):

_____

_____

Questions that should have been included:

_____

_____

Questions that should be eliminated:

_____

_____

Design and user friendliness of the instrument:

_____

_____

Other:

_____

_____

FORM FOR INTERVIEWING FAMILY MEMBER

Name of client_____Date of interview_____

Person interviewed_____

Relationship to client_____

Age _____S/M/D_____

Spouse's name _____ Age _____

Children _____

If sibling, place in birth order:

_____

Was there anything unusual about the gestation or birth of client? Y / N If yes, please describe:

_____

_____

_____

_____

_____

_____

What was client like as a child?

_____

_____

_____

_____

_____

_____

_____

Did client have any unusual behavior or behavior problems? Y / N If yes, please describe:

_____

_____

_____

_____

_____

_____

How were client and siblings disciplined?

_____

_____

_____

_____

_____

_____

Did client have any learning problems? Y / N If yes, please describe:

_____

_____

_____

_____

_____

_____

_____

_____

What was your relationship like with client when he/she was a child?

_____

_____

_____

_____

_____

_____

Do you recall the onset of client's mental illness? If yes, what were the circumstances?

_____

_____

_____

_____

_____

What types of symptoms did client have at that time (hallucinations, delusions, etc.)?

_____

_____

_____

_____

_____

_____

_____

_____

Are you familiar with the treatment or services client has received since onset? If yes, what do you think has been most effective?

_____

_____

_____

_____

_____

_____

Have you been involved with client's treatment or are you currently? If yes, please describe involvement:

_____

_____

_____

_____

_____

_____

If client is agreeable, would you like to be involved in treatment through our program? Y / N and/or have more information regarding services provided to client by our CSP? Y / N If yes, please specify:

_____

_____

_____

_____

_____

_____

_____

_____

Are you familiar with client's past and present medications? Y / N If yes, which do you feel have been most effective and what concerns do you have regarding medications?

_____

_____

_____

_____

_____

Does client have any AODA issues past or present? Y / N Has he received treatment? Y / N If yes, specify:

_____

_____

_____

_____

_____

_____

_____

Do any other family members (extended and immediate) have AODA issues? Y / N If yes, please specify:

_____

_____

_____

_____

_____

_____

_____

Do any other family members (immediate and extended) have mental health problems? If yes, please specify who, nature of problem, and treatment:

_____

_____

_____

_____

_____

_____

_____

_____

_____

_____

Do any family members have significant health problems? Y / N If yes, specify:

_____

_____

_____

_____

_____

_____

_____

_____

_____

_____

Has client ever been verbally/physically/sexually abusive towards you? Y / N If yes, specify (dates, circumstances, number of incidents, perceived relation to person's mental illness):

_____

_____

_____

_____

_____

Was there any incident of physical/verbal/sexual abuse involving any other family members? If yes, specify:

_____

_____

_____

_____

_____

How often do you see or talk with client?

_____

_____

_____

_____

_____

Who initiates contact?

_____

_____

Would you like to see client more/less often? Under different circumstances? Specify:

_____

_____

What is the nature of your interaction during contact?

_____

_____

_____

_____

Do you assist client with any routine daily activities? Y / N If yes, specify:

_____

_____

_____

_____

When you have contact with client, what types of symptoms do you notice?

_____

_____

_____

_____

_____

How do you respond to them? What seems to work best for you in your responses?

_____

_____

_____

_____

_____

Siblings

Name_____ Age_____ Marital (S/M/D/W) _____

Occupation _____ Residence_____

Name_____ Age_____ Marital (S/M/D/W) _____

Occupation _____ Residence_____

Name_____ Age_____ Marital (S/M/D/W) _____

Occupation _____ Residence_____

Name_____ Age_____ Marital (S/M/D/W) _____

Occupation _____ Residence_____

Is parents' marriage intact? Y / N / NA _____

Married how many years_____

History of residence (where family has lived, reason for moves, client's reaction to moves):

_____

_____

_____

_____

_____

_____

Client's special talents:

_____

_____

_____

_____

_____

_____

Is client able to talk with you about his/her mental illness? Y / N If not, why do you think he/she is unable?

_____

_____

_____

_____

_____

_____

_____

Are you familiar with the Alliance for the Mentally Ill? Y / N If yes, do you receive their newsletter? Y / N Attend meetings? Y / N If you are not familiar with AMI, would you like information about it? Y / N Would you like any additional information about mental illness or resources for families? Y / N Specify:

_____

_____

_____

_____

_____

_____

_____

How do you think the CSP can help your relative?

_____

_____

_____

_____

_____

Additional Questions for Offspring

When did you realize your parent had a mental illness?

_____

_____

Did you ever spend time in foster care or live with someone other than your parent? Y / N If yes, please specify:

_____

_____

_____

Was your parent ever verbally/physically/sexually abusive toward you? Y / N If yes, specify:

_____

_____

_____

_____

How would you describe your relationship with your parent when you were a child?

_____

_____

_____

_____

What is it like now?

_____

_____

_____

_____

Would you like to see your parent more/less? Specify:

_____

_____

_____

_____

_____

Did you receive counseling/support while you were growing up to help you deal with your parent's mental illness? Y / N Specify:

_____

_____

_____

_____

Do you have information about the causes of mental illness? Y / N If no, would you like some? Y / N

_____

_____

Other information:

_____

_____

_____

_____

_____

Person completing this interview _____

FORM FOR INTERVIEWING SIGNIFICANT OTHERS

Client name _____ Date of interview _____

Person interviewed _____ Age _____

Nature of relationship_____

How long have you known client? _____

How did you meet?

_____

_____

_____

_____

_____

_____

What do you know about his/her mental illness?

_____

_____

_____

_____

_____

_____

How often to you see and talk with client?

_____

_____

Who initiates contact?

_____

What do you do together?

_____

_____

_____

_____

Do you assist client with routine daily tasks? Y / N If yes, specify:

_____

_____

_____

What types of symptoms do you notice when client is with you? Are they different from symptoms that you have noticed in the past?

_____

_____

_____

_____

Does client have any unusual behaviors? Y / N If yes, describe:

_____

_____

_____

Has client ever been verbally or physically abusive towards you? Y / N If yes, specify:

_____

_____

_____

_____

Are you familiar with client' past/present treatment and services? Y / N If yes, have you been involved in any way? Y / N Specify:

_____

_____

_____

_____

_____

What do you think has been beneficial?

_____

_____

_____

_____

_____

If client is agreeable, would you like to be involved in treatment Y / N and/or have more information about services provided to client by CSP? Y / N

_____

_____

_____

_____

_____

Does client have any AODA issues that you are aware of? Y /N If yes, specify (nature, treatment, etc.):

_____

_____

_____

_____

_____

Would you like to see client more/less often? Specify:

_____

_____

_____

_____

_____

How do you think the CSP can help client?

_____

_____

_____

_____

_____

What do you believe are client's strengths and weaknesses?

_____

_____

_____

_____

_____

Additional comments:

_____

_____

_____

_____

Person completing this interview _____

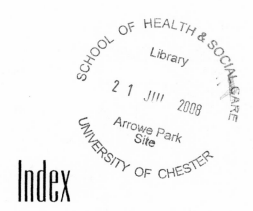

Index